Meat Hygiene and Fresh Meat Technology

NIPA® GENX ELECTRONIC RESOURCES & SOLUTIONS P. LTD.
New Delhi-110 034

About the Authors

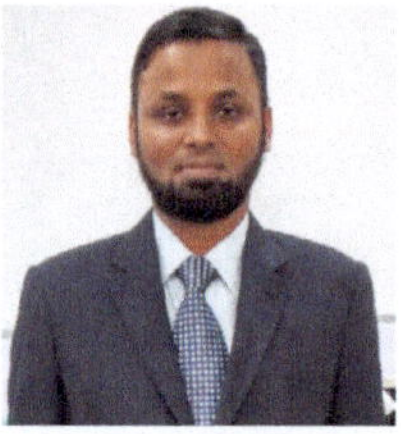

Dr. Tanbir Ahmad was born in a village called Hasanpur Surat, Shahpur Patory, District Samastipur, State Bihar, India in 1980. He did his secondary and senior secondary schooling from Jawahar Navodaya Vidyalaya (JNV), Samastipur, Bihar, India. He obtained his Bachelor's degree in Veterinary Science from Madras Veterinary College, (under Tamil Nadu Veterinary and Animal Sciences University, Chennai, Tamil Nadu), Chennai, India in 2005. He got his Master degree in Livestock Products Technology from Bihar Veterinary College Patna, Bihar, India in 2008. In November 2009, he joined Indian Council of Agricultural Research (ICAR), New Delhi, India as Scientist. He did his Ph.D Degree in 2018 from Universiti Putra Malaysia, Malaysia as in-service candidate by availing ICAR-International Fellowship from Indian Council of Agricultural Research, New Delhi, India. He is recipient of Best Ph.D Thesis Award (2018) from Faculty of Agriculture, Universiti Putra Malaysia, Malaysia, Best Employee Award in the category of Best in Publication (2018) from ICAR-Central Institute of Post-Harvest Engineering & Technology, Ludhiana, Punjab, India and ICAR-Senior Research Fellowship (PGS)-2009 with Fellowship in Livestock Products Technology from ICAR, New Delhi, India. At present, he is working as Senior Scientist at ICAR-Indian Veterinary Research Institute (IVRI), Bareilly, UP, India.

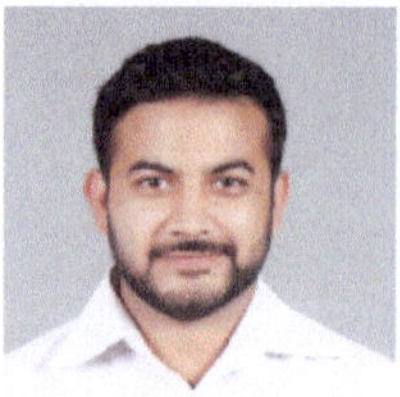

Dr. Suman Talukder, born in 1982, started his carrier as Scientist in the Division of Livestock Products Technology, ICAR-IVRI, Izatnagar, in 2010. He completed his Ph.D. in Livestock Products Technology, from the ICAR-IVRI, Bareilly, UP in 2018. Dr. Suman Talukder has expertise in the field of meat products development, animal byproducts technology and packaging of livestock derived foods. He has published more than 64 research articles and 17 book chapters. Dr. Suman Talukder has vast experience in teaching undergraduate and post-graduate students in the subject of Livestock Products Technology. Presently, he is working as Senior Scientist in the Division of Livestock Products Technology ICAR-IVRI, Bareilly, UP, India-243122.

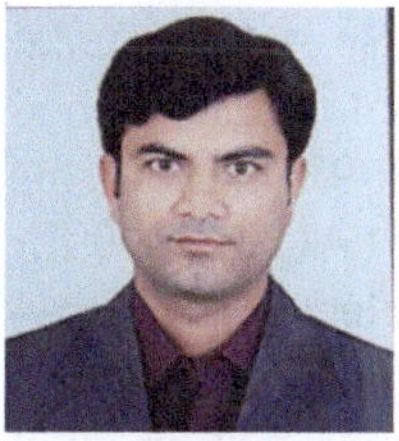

Dr. Devendra Kumar was born in 1980 in Saran, Bihar. He completed his graduation in Veterinary Science and Animal Husbandry (B.V.Sc. & A.H) from College of Veterinary and Animal Science, Khanapara, Guwahati in 2005, M.V.Sc. (2007) in Livestock Products Technology (LPT) from Govind Ballabh Pant University of Agriculture and Technology, Pantnagar and Ph.D in Livestock Products Technology (LPT) from Guru Angad Dev Veterinary and Animal Sciences University, Ludhiana in 2016. He joined Indian Council of Agricultural Research (ICAR) in 2009 as Scientist and served at ICAR-National Research Centre on Camel, Bikaner from 2010 to 2019 and presently working as Senior Scientist in LPT Division of ICAR-IVRI, Izatnagar, Bareilly. Dr. Kumar has work experience in meat/dairy science, food safety, protein/peptide and health oriented meat/milk products processing. Dr. Kumar has published several research articles in reputed National and International Journals including Popular Articles, Book Chapters and many research papers abstracts in National/ International Scientific Seminars and Conferences.

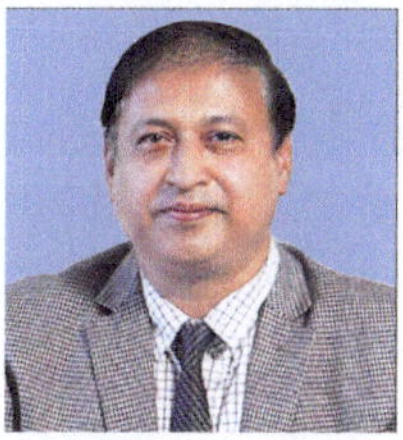

Dr. Arup Ratan Sen was born at Biur, Bankura, West Bengal in 1968. He is the graduate of Bidhan Chandra Krishi Viswavidyalaya, Nadia, West Bengal. He obtained his Master and Ph.D degrees in Livestock Products Technology from Livestock Products Technology Division of ICAR-Indian Veterinary Research Institute, Izatnagar, UP-243122. Dr. Arup Ratan Sen, in his career spanning about 28 years has contributed exclusively in the area of meat production, processing, value addition and quality control of meat and meat products. He has handled 8 extramural research projects worth 8.21 crores both as PI and Co-PI funded by NAIP (World bank), MoFPI, DAC *etc.* in the last 10 years. He had developed technologies for hygienic slaughtering of food animals, value added meat products, packaging, shelf-life enhancement. He has undergone training under DBT-Overseas Fellowship at Danish Institute of Agricultural Sciences, Denmark on state-of the art "Implications of animal genomes on meat quality", studied the pig gene and pork quality and developed meat genomic lab at NRC on Meat. He has successfully completed a couple of sponsored research project funded by Industries and involved with many success stories. He serves as Editor Journal of Meat Science and Guest Editor, Indian Journal of Animal Health. He has published 4 books, 8 book chapters and more than 80 research publications in the National and International Journal of repute and he has been conferred with DBT, NAVS, IMSA fellowships and other National and Scientific Society awards. Currently, he is holding the post of Head, Division of Livestock Products Technology, ICAR-Indian Veterinary Research Institute Izatnagar, Bareilly, UP.

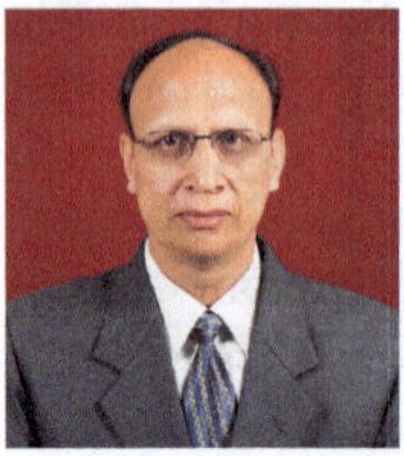

Dr. S. K. Mendiratta completed his M.V.Sc. (gold medal 1990) and Ph.D in Livestock Products Technology and joined as a scientist at ICAR-IVRI, Izatnagar in 1992. Due to his outstanding research work, he got selected by FAO in 2000 for training in the USA. Again in 2005, he was selected by INSA-DFG for training in Germany. Dr. S.K. Mendiratta has expertise in the field of various meat quality improvement, new product development and animal byproducts technology. With experience of more than 32 years in the field of Livestock Products Technology, he has developed more than 17 new technologies, published more than 158 research papers and authored many books. Dr. S.K. Mendiratta received best teacher awards and was associated with many organizations of national and international repute in the field. He has vast experience in teaching undergraduate and post-graduate students in the subject of Livestock Products Technology. Presently, he is serving as the Joint Director (Academic) at ICAR-IVRI, Deemed University, Izatnagar, Bareilly, UP, India.

Meat Hygiene and Fresh Meat Technology

Tanbir Ahmad
Senior Scientist
Division of Livestock Products Technology
ICAR-Indian Veterinary Research Institute
Izatnagar, Bareilly-243122, Uttar Pradesh, India

Suman Talukder
Senior Scientist
Division of Livestock Products Technology
ICAR-Indian Veterinary Research Institute
Izatnagar, Bareilly-243122, Uttar Pradesh, India

Devendra Kumar
Senior Scientist
Division of Livestock Products Technology
ICAR-Indian Veterinary Research Institute
Izatnagar, Bareilly-243122, Uttar Pradesh, India

Arup Ratan Sen
Head
Division of Livestock Products Technology
ICAR-Indian Veterinary Research Institute
Izatnagar, Bareilly-243122, Uttar Pradesh, India

S. K. Mendiratta
Joint Director (Academics)
ICAR-Indian Veterinary Research Institute
Izatnagar, Bareilly-243122, Uttar Pradesh, India

nipa®

NIPA® GENX ELECTRONIC RESOURCES & SOLUTIONS P. LTD.
New Delhi-110 034

NIPA® GENX ELECTRONIC RESOURCES & SOLUTIONS P. LTD.

101,103, Vikas Surya Plaza, CU Block
L.S.C. Market, Pitam Pura, New Delhi-110 034
Ph : +91-11-43860225, Mob.: +91 9717133558, 9540816132
E-mail: newindiapublishingagency@gmail.com
Website: www.nipaersources.com

Print ISBN: 978-93-58876-16-1
ebook ISBN: 978-93-58874-97-6

NIPA® also publishes books in a variety of electronic formats. Some content that appears in print may not be available in electronic books, and vice versa.

Composed and Designed by NIPA®.

Preface

Meat science sits at the intersection of animal biology, public health, engineering, and food technology. This book has been developed to give students and practitioners a coherent, step-by-step understanding of how live animals become safe, high-quality meat—anchored in scientific principles and grounded in practical realities of modern slaughterhouses.

We begin Chapter 1 by introducing meat animals and the scope of the sector, establishing terminology and the diversity of species and production systems. Chapter 2 builds the biological foundation with meat animal anatomy and the composition of meat, linking structure to function and, ultimately, to product quality.

The transition from farm to abattoir is addressed holistically. Chapter 3 details slaughterhouse layout and essential facilities, emphasizing product flow, worker safety, and regulatory compliance. Chapter 4 explores transportation and handling, demonstrating how stress physiology and welfare outcomes translate directly into measurable meat quality traits. Pre- and post-slaughter health safeguards are covered in Chapters 5 and 6, where ante-mortem and post-mortem examination procedures are presented as complementary pillars of food safety, disease control, and carcass judgment.

The core technical operations are treated comprehensively in Chapter 7, outlining humane slaughtering methods, hygienic dressing, and critical control points. Because sustainability and value recovery are central to modern meat plants, Chapter 8 highlights the utilization of slaughterhouse by-products, turning potential waste into edible, pharmaceutical, and industrial resources.

A strong scientific backbone underpins quality management. Chapters 9–11 unpack muscle structure, the molecular basis of contraction–relaxation, and muscle protein composition—equipping readers to connect biochemistry with texture, water-holding capacity, and color. Chapter 12 explains post-mortem (anaerobic) glycolysis and the cascade of biochemical changes that define ultimate pH and eating quality. Building on this, Chapter 13 presents conditioning and tenderization strategies—ageing, mechanical and enzymatic options—so practitioners can select evidence-based interventions.

Product preservation and safety engineering are addressed in Chapter 14, covering storage of fresh meat, cold-chain management, microbial ecology, and shelf-life optimization. The basics of meat physiochemical properties are dealt extensively in Chapter 15 so as to provide comprehensive knowledge about effects of these properties on the overall quality of meat . Meat plant hygiene receives focused treatment in Chapter 16, with actionable guidance on cleaning, sanitation, and hygienic design to prevent contamination and cross-contamination. Recognizing environmental stewardship as non-negotiable, Chapter 17 explains the working of effluent treatment plants, linking compliance to sustainable operations.

Throughout, we have aimed for clarity, practicality, and alignment with contemporary standards in animal welfare, hazard analysis and critical control points (HACCP), and environmental compliance. Figures, tables, and process flows (where provided in the full text) are designed to support rapid learning and on-floor application.

This volume is intended for undergraduate and postgraduate students in veterinary, animal science, and food technology; for inspectors and quality professionals; and for managers and engineers seeking a concise yet rigorous reference. We hope it serves both as a textbook and a day-to-day guide to safer, more efficient, and more sustainable meat production.

The authors are thankful to Dr. Triveni Dutt, Director cum Vice Chancellor, Dr. Sanjay Kumar Singh (Joint Director, Research) and Dr. S. K. Mendiratta, Joint Director (Academic) of the premier institute, ICAR-IVRI, Bareilly, UP, India for providing the necessary support for the publication of the book.

Suggestions for betterment and corrections are most welcome from teachers, scientists and students.

Authors

Contents

1

Introduction to Meat Animals

Introduction

Generally, muscles and offals obtained from animals feeding on grass and various other cultivated crops are regarded as meat. Apart from the meat obtained from the cattle, sheep, goat, pig and poultry, in many countries particularly Denmark, Belgium, Holland and Germany, horse meat is also consumed (hippophasia) as normal meat. Kangaroos are slaughtered for meat in Australia whereas capybara a large semi-aquatic vegetarian rodent, is used in South America as of one of the meat source. Dog meat (fragrant) is relished (Kinophasia) in few cultures such as South Korea, China, Vietnam and few north eastern states of India.

In many parts of the world including Indian subcontinent, buffalo meat (*Bubalus bubalis*), also known as water buffalo or arna, is quite popular owing to its tenderness, leanness and low cholesterol qualities. It is distributed in many countries around the world such as India (largest population), Pakistan, China, Bangladesh, Indonesia, Philippines, Hungary, Italy and France *etc.* Bison (*Bison bison*) from North America is also called buffalo but they are separate species of the order Bovidae. Rabbits are also source of meat having higher growth rate and better feed conversion ratio (2:1). Elands are another meat source which are raised in Africa and Russia for meat purpose.

Meat is quite high in protein content but the presence of saturated fat is perceived negatively due to its association in various cardiovascular diseases, diabetes *etc.* Efforts are made to produce lean meat having higher content of unsaturated fatty acids and to reduce the ω-6 to ω -3 fatty acids ratio.

Large ruminants meat breeds

- Aberdeen-Angus – best beef breed
- In UK, Friesian is the dominant dairy breed (80%)
- 55% of the beef is produced from dairy breed in Uinted Kingdom
- Hereford and Aberdeen Angus beef breeds are used to produce beef cattle.

- French Charolais is large cattle breed having rapid growth rate and lean meat.
- Luing was developed from cross of Shorthorn and Highland Cattle
- Main European beef breeds are Simmental and Friesian
- Droughtmaster cattle has been developed from Zebu or Brahman (*Bos Indicus*) with British beef breeds (Shorthorns and Hereford) (*Bos taurus*)
- *Bos Indicus*—disease resistance and hardiness
- *Bos Taurus*— productivity and early maturity

Systems of large ruminants meat production

i. Range system
ii. Semi-intensive system
iii. Intensive system
    - Demand is for lean meat with minimum fat covering, tender, palatable and relatively cheap
    - So, slaughter animal of age 15 to 24 months
    - Bulls carcase is 10% heavier, meat is leaner, 12% faster growth rate and 8% higher feed conversion than steers
    - But bull beef is darker cutting appearance, lacks finish, shows 'bullish' characteristics and lacks continuity of supply
    - Young bull beef is differentiated by inferior quality beef from old bull by the much darker colour of the later meat
    - Bobby calves have low muscle to bone ratio and hence loss to consumer
    - Fatstock—livestock raised with such a feeding so that to have a lot of fat deposits around the meat
    - Leanstock/ meat—stock-livestock raised to have lean meat

Barley beef system

Specific system of meat production where early weaning of calves are done and then raised on *ad lib* concentrate till the slaughter age of 11 months attaining 400 kg weight and feed conversion ratio of 5.5.

Meat analogue ---is soya protein spun into filaments and bound with more protein such as egg albumin.

Textured vegetable protein--- meals, concentrates or protein isolates combined with carbohydrates in the form of starch or carageenan by extrusion at high pressure at 115-175 °C.

Extended meat--- is a mixture of vegetable and meat protein which is subjected to normal heat processing. Various colours, flavours and even fat can be added.

World livestock production

World produced 361 million tonnes of meat by slaughtering almost 90 billion animals in 2022 out of which poultry meat production was 138 million tonnes. The largest volume of share is taken by poultry meat followed by pork, beef and mutton. In general, those countries with the highest meat consumption rates are also the major producers. In 2024, Brazil was the largest beef exporter globally and other major beef exporters were Australia, the United States, India, Argentina and New Zealand. China is the largest importer of meat in 2023 followed by the United States of America, South Korea, Japan and Italy.

Status of meat production in India

Globally, India has got the largest livestock population (Basic Animal Husbandry Statistics (BAHS), 2024, 20th Livestock Census. Department of Animal Husbandry and Dairying, Ministry of Fisheries, Animal Husbandry & Dairying, Government of India) of around 535.78 million as per the 20th Livestock Census, 2019. Among this, 109.85 million is contributed by buffalo population (BAHS, 2020). As per the 19th Livestock Census, the buffalo population was showing an increase of 1.1%. Uttar Pradesh, Rajasthan and Gujarat are the leading states in India for buffalo population (BAHS, 2020). Uttar Pradesh contributes 33 million, Rajasthan 13.7 million and Gujarat contributes 10.5 million buffaloes (BAHS, 2020). In India, the total meat production is 10.25 million tonnes reflecting a 4.95% growth over 2022-23, out of which buffalo, goat, sheep and poultry meat shares are 1.854 (18.08%), 1.588 (15.49%), 1.141 (11.13%) and 5.019 (48.49%) million tonnes, respectively (BAHS, 2024). India's global ranking in meat production is fourth. The major meat production contributing states are West Bengal (12.62%) followed by Uttar Pradesh (12.29%) and Maharashtra (11.28%) (BAHS, 2024). Such a huge quantity of meat production came from slaughtering of 13.62 million buffalo, 80.70 million sheep, 135.17 million goats, 0.96 million pigs and 3354.97 million poultry during the year 2023-24 (BAHS, 2024).

Uttar Pradesh is the second top producer of meat among the Indian states having share of 12.29% of total national meat production and it has registered a growth rate of 5.69% in meat production during the period 2023-24 (Basic Animal Husbandry Statistics, 2024). Uttar Pradesh produced 361.33, 81.50 and 8.94 thousand tonnes of poultry, goat and sheep meat, respectively in 2023-24 placing it 7th, 8th and 11th among the Indian states in poultry, goat and sheep meat production, respectively (Basic Animal Husbandry Statistics, 2024).

India is the third-largest producer of broiler meat in the world producing nearly 5.02 million ton in 2023-24 and Uttar Pradesh share in the national chicken meat production is 36.13 thousand MT which is nearly 7.19%. There are 148.88 and 74.26 millions of goat and sheep, respectively in India out of which approximately 144.80 and 9.85 lakhs of goat and sheep, respectively are in Uttar Pradesh production (Basic Animal Husbandry Statistics, 2024). Corresponding number of goats and sheep slaughtered during the same period was reported to be 55.53 and 5.96 lakhs, respectively.

Hormone growth promoters

- Growth before puberty is largely controlled by growth hormone (GH)
- In males, body tissue and organs growth is stimulated by androgens
- Early maturation of muscles and bones is brought by anabolic oestrogens
- Growth promoting substances are mainly used to ward off the negative impact of castration on body growth
- Natural growth hormone implant for heifer --- 200 mg of testosterone propionate and 20 mg of oestradiol benzoate given as eight pellets to animals 180 kg or more. Given as subcutaneous injection in ear
- Diethylstilboestrol is illegally used in veal calf production

Probiotics

- Probiotics are harmless bacteria provided orally to young animals at early stage of life and bacteria get established in GI tract
- The probiotics are said to be helpful in enhancing feed conversion efficiency, and maintain animal health and thus, ensures early slaughter age

Prebiotics

- Compounds that are administered orally along with other food resulting in higher body growth and/or enhanced favourable effects on intestinal microbes.

Definitions related to cattle

- Bull: An uncastrated male bovine
- Heifer: A female bovine till the first calving
- Cow: A female bovine having one or more calving
- Steer or bullock: A male castrated early in life (at 6–12 weeks old)
- Stag: A male castrated later in life having well developed body confirmation compared to the bullock
- Bobby calves: calves slaughtered within few days of birth

Sheep

- Sheep were the first animal domesticated by man
- Two breeds namely Finnish Landrace and Russian Romanov are known for producing three lambs/ewe/year

Sheep farming systems: Two

i. Hill sheep farming system

- These sheep are small, hardy and thrifty in nature possessing long wool
- They attain late maturity and low in fecundity
- Breeds included in this system are: North Country Cheviot, South Country Cheviot, Scottish Blackface, Welsh Mountain, Derbyshire Gritstone and Lonk
- The number of sheep raised under this system is higher than the lowland farming

ii. Lowland sheep farming system

- These sheep are early maturing, having short wool, higher carcase weights and high in fecundity
- Suffolk, Dorset Horn and Dorset Down, Southdown and Shropshire are the main lowland breeds
- Merinos are predominant sheep breed (75%) in Australia whereas Romney Marsh is the main breed in New Zealand followed by Corriedales, Merinos and Southdowns and their crosses
- Rambouillet is the major sheep breed in the United States
- In eastern Mediterranean and Iraq, Awassi sheep breed is the chief coarse wool type sheep-- wool is used for making carpets
- Cashmere and mohair sheep breeds are known for fine sheep wools. However, fine qulity fibre are also obtained from Angora goats and rabbits, alpacas and llamas
- Technically, 'mutton' is the meat obtained from pre-weaned lambs and not from ewes, wethers, hoggets and rams
- Good mutton breed qualities should have short plump neck, flesh full chest, wide breast and shoulder with ribs full of flesh, wide full back, short stocky plump legs, thick full loin
- Aberdeen angus- best beef breed (60% carcase yield)
- Suffolk- best mutton breed (50% Carcase yield)
- Mandya - from Karnatka--- best mutton breed in India

Definitions

- Lamb: A sheep from birth to weaning time (generally at 3½–4½ months old). According to butchers --- a sheep from birth until shearing time the following year (a sheep 13 months old is still classed as lamb)
- Hogget: A 'lamb'in its second year of its life having two permanent incisor teeth
- Tup or ram: The uncastrated male sheep
- Wether: The castrated male
- Gimmer: A female sheep not given birth to any lamb
- Ewe: A female sheep which has given birth to lambs
- Cast ewe: Female sheep which is no longer used for breeding

Pigs

- Large White, Landrace, Duroc, Hampshire and Piétrain are the prominent commercial breeds
- In old boars, oval shaped cartilage over the shoulder area becomes calcified which is known as 'shield'

Glossary of terms

- Boar: Matured male pig used for breeding
- Gilt: A matured female used for breeding just before furrowing
- Pig: Male or female pigs of any age used for fattening or breeding
- Piglet: A pig till the age of weaning
- Rearing pig: A pig from 10 weeks to slaughter or service
- Sow: A female after the first farrowing
- Weaner: A pig from weaning to the age of 10 weeks
- Stag: A male pig castrated late in life to enhance fattening and prevent the boar odour
- Rig: A male pig with only one descended testicle in scrotum

Classes of pigs

Pork pigs

- Live weight of 54-63 kg at 14-18 weeks
- Dead weight of 39-45 kg with a dressing % of 70-72
- Carcases are graded as Q, A and B based on back fat thickness (45, 65 and 80 mm, respectively)

Cutter pig

- Live weight of 45-63 kg at 18-24 weeks
- Dead weight of 63-82 kg having dressing percentage of 72-75
- These are heavier pork pigs
- Grading same as above

Bacon pigs

- Live weight of 84-93 kg at 22-28 weeks of age
- Dead weight of 61-70 kg
- Dressing % -- 75
- Bacon, hams and other smoked products are prepared
- Four grades based on back fat thickness

Heavy pigs

- Live weight of 100-114 kg at 26-34 weeks of age
- Dead weight of 75-88 kg
- Dressing % --- 78-80%

Goats

- Meat with low saturated fat content
- Goat breeds from which hair are obtained- Angora and Cashmere
- Chief foreign goat breeds- Alpine, Toggenburg and Nubian
- Black Bengal—best goat meat breed in India

Poultry

Definitions

- *Broilers:* Fast growing poultry slaughtered at around 42 days with FCR of 1.75 and of around 2.3 kg live weight
- *Poussins:* 23–28 days old retail sold young poultry birds having 0.5 kg live weight with dressed weight of 0.25–5 kg
- *Paté de foie gras:* is a delicacy prepared from fat liver of geese who are force-fed with noodles or other foods so as to cause fatty liver (enlargement of liver).
- *Hens:* Female which have passed its laying stage
- *Capons:* Castrated male bird (live weight of 3 kg)

Rabbits

- The Commercial breeds of rabbit are New Zealand White and Californian
- The optimum slaughter weight -- around 2.7 kg at 12–14 weeks of age
- Rabbit meat is low in fat (3.8%) and high in protein (20.7%) which is comparable with chicken meat which has 2.5% fat and 21.5% protein
- Feed conversion efficiency 2.5 : 1
- Stunning is by electricity

Deer

- Deer farming is popular in United Kingdom and other European countries and is done on huge scale in New Zealand
- Dear meat called venison is quite lean, low in fat (5–10%) which is quite lower than beef and lamb (25–40% fat)
- Slaughtering age -- 8–30 months and produce dressed carcase weights of 53–60 kg

2

Meat Animal Anatomy and Composition of Meat

- The proportion of bone varies depending on breed and body condition from 12 to 28% in the dressed carcase and approximately 15% in a good large ruminants carcase
- Bone percentage increases with the age and weight of the animal and it is lowest in Aberdeen Angus cattle and it may increase to 28% in low quality large ruminants
- The average bone % in bobby calves is 50%, veal calves 25%, in lamb 17–35%, in pork 12–20% and in poultry 8–17%

Important parts of digestive system of meat animals

Ox tongue

- Filiform papillae found on the tongue are pointing backward and horny and thus, helps in food prehension
- Actinobacillosis erodes the prominent posterior part of the tongue dorsum
- 10–14 circumvallate papillae are spread in the region of prominent dorsum around the either side of the tongue midline
- Black pigmentation of the tongue surface is fairly normal and not associated with any disease condition

Sheep and goat tongue

- Similar to cattle tongue
- However, papillae are not horny but the centre of the tip is slightly grooved
- Black pigmentation of the surface of the tongue is common in black-skinned sheep.

Pig tongue

- It is narrow and long but devoid of dorsal ridge
- Base of the tongue shows one or two circumvallate papillae on each side of the tongue midline whereas fungiform papillae are spread throughout the whole surface

Horse tongue

- It is flat and long ending in spatula shape
- Dorsal ridge is absent and on each side of the tongue one circumvallate papilla is present
- The epiglottis is pointed
- Pigmentation is always absent

Stomach

Ox stomach

- Rumen, reticulum, omasum and abomasum are the four compartments of the stomach or paunch occupying 150 litres of volume
- 75% of the abdominal cavity is occupied by rumen
- Abomasum acts as the real stomach as it secretes the gastric juice
- The omasum and abomasum are connected by omentum or caul fat with the posterior part of the liver

Mucous membranes of stomach of ox

- *Rumen:* May be black or brown in colour excluding on pillars or folds which appear pale having presence of large papillae
- *Reticulum:* Has honeycomb-like look studded with cells of sides 4, 5 or 6
- *Omasum:* Also known as 'bible' having about 100 distinct longitudinal folds
- *Abomasum:* True stomach possessing distinct oblique folds (almost 30 in number) which is absent in the pyloric region

Sheep and goat stomach

In Scotland, the sheep rumen is used as container for **haggis** (sheep stomach stuffed with cooked sheep pluck (minced heart, liver and lungs) added with seasoning ingredients such as chopped onion mixed with oatmeal, salt, pepper, cayenne, nutmeg and grated beef suet)

Liver

Ox

- The largest gland in the body
- It weighs almost 1% of the live weight averaging 5.4 kg

Pig

- Pig liver has five lobes
- Look like '***Morocco leather***' because of the presence of considerable observable interlobular tissue

Horse

Gall bladder is absent

Pancreas

- Is also called gut sweetbread
- Insulin and glucagon is released by the Islet of Langerhans

Lungs

Ox lungs

The left lung is three lobed and 4 to 5 lobes are found in right lung

Horse lungs

- Have 2 lobes in left lung and 3 lobes in right lungs

Pluck

- It consists of larynx, trachea, lungs, heart and liver in case of large ruminants, sheep, goat and calf
- Oesophagus is also included in case of pig pluck
- In pig- trachea has 32 cartilaginous rings
- In sheep- trachea has about 50 rings

Spleen (melt)

- Spleen is also called melt
- Not indispensable
- This organ is the site of breakdown of old red cells and platelets as well as storage place of RBCs

Lymphatic system

- In ox, the mesenteric lymph nodes are black in colour whereas in the pig, these are lobulated and white except the lymph nodes of the head and neck which are red in colour

Important lymph node

Haemal lymph nodes

- Pea sized, oval lymph nodes varying in colour from dark red to roughly black having no afferent and efferent lymphatics
- Also called accessory spleens
- In the ox and sheep, haemal lymph nodes are found abundantly in number whereas these are absent in the horse and pig
- Found particularly in the subcutaneous fat and along the route of aorta in cattle
- Normally found under the peritoneum in the sublumbar area in sheep, lamb and goat and it becomes enlarged and more in number in animals affected with anaemia and cachectic conditions

Lymph nodes of head and neck

i. Submaxillary lymph node
ii. Parotid lymph node
iii. Retropharyngeal lymph node

Prescapular lymph node

- Significant for detection of bovine tuberculosis
- Its drainage area includes head, neck, shoulder and forelimb as well as the muscle and bone
- If tuberculous lesions are detected in prescapular node and not found in the head or its lymph nodes, it clearly indicates the infection of the lymph node is due to local inoculation or spread through blood

Inspector' node

- Located at the joint of the two cardiac lobes of the right lung and are present in 75% of cattle carcase

Splenic lymph nodes

- These are not found in the ox and sheep

Popliteal lymph node

- Not found in 50% carcase and present superficially
- A small subcutaneous node, known as the **hock node or Hartenstein's gland** is the small subcutaneous node present in all cases and is situated superficially a hand's width above the tuber calcis on the posterior side of the limb

Urogenital system

Kidneys

Ox kidneys

- Lobulated (10-25 lobes) and reddish brown in colour
- Left kidney is mobile and position of right kidney is fixed

Sheep and goat kidneys

- Bean shaped kidneys are dark brown and not lobulated

Pig kidneys

- Bean –shaped, reddish brown kidneys with smooth surfaces

Horse kidneys

- The shape of left kidney is bean like whereas the right kidney is heart or triangular-shaped

Endocrine system

Thymus gland

- The true sweetbread having pinkish white in colour and lobulated
- It is found in two regions;
  - i. The gland situated in the thoracic cavity and rich in fat--- **heart bread**
  - ii. The gland situated in the neck region and constituted of two lobes--- **neck bread**

Horns

- Useful in determining the age of cattle
- Small wrinkles found at the base of the horns are not to be counted because such rings indicate poor feeding of animal during the growth period
- The first ring is formed at around 2 years of age and subsequently one ring is added annually
- So, age of the animal is the total number of rings present on the horn plus one

Muscular system

- The muscular system is composed of
  - Skeletal—which are striated and voluntary in nature
  - Cardiac —which are striated and involuntary in nature and
  - Smooth —which are non-striated and involuntary in nature --- found in certain organs, glands and blood vessels

- 25–45% of the live weight of the animal is made of skeletal muscles
- Animal body has approximately 300 muscles

Fat

- 'Marbling' is the deposition of fat between the muscle fibres
- Marbling takes place in well fed young animals and not in older animals in which fat deposits subcutaneously
- 'Marbling' is not encountered in horses
- Value of edible fat ranks second only to the hide/skin in value
- 'Baloon kidneys'-- abnormal amount of kidney fat
- Industrially, oleo oil and oleo stearin are obtained from edible fat to manufacture margarine
- Oleo stearin is also used to solidify the cooking fat and for soap and candle making
- Whereas inedible fat is utilized to manufacture soap, lubricants, candles and glycerine as well used as a binder in animal feed preparations

Determination of age by dentition

Table 2.1: Dental formula for the ox, sheep and goat

		Incisor	Canine	Premolar	Molar	Total
Temporary (deciduous) teeth	Upper	0	0	3	-	20
	Lower	3	1	3	-	
Permanent teeth	Upper	0	0	3	3	32
	Lower	3	1	3	3	

Table 2.2: Dental formula for the pig

		Incisor	Canine	Premolar	Molar	Total
Temporary (deciduous) teeth	Upper	3	1	3	-	28
	Lower	3	1	3	-	
Permanent teeth	Upper	3	1	4	3	44
	Lower	3	1	4	3	

Table 2.3: Dental formula for the horse

		Incisor	Canine	Premolar	Molar	Total
Temporary (deciduous) teeth	Upper	3	0	3	-	24
	Lower	3	0	3	-	
Permanent teeth	Upper	3	1	3 (4)	3	40
	Lower	3	1	3	3	(42)

Determination of age by horn

- Based on counting the number of horn rings
- Wrinkles found at the base of the horn is indication of lack of nutrition during the growth

Determination of sex of dressed carcase

Bull

- Open external inguinal ring is found partially covered by little amount of scrotal fat
- Well developed bulbocavernosus muscle (also called erector and refractor penis muscle)
- Gracilis muscle -- triangular shaped
- Meat of young bull --- light/brick red
- Whereas meat from older bull--- dark red, dry and little fat content

Table 2.4: Differentiation of sheep and goat carcases

S. No.	Features	Sheep	Goat
1	Back & withers	round & well fleshed	Sharp, little flesh
2	Thorax	barrel-shaped	Flattened laterally
3	Tail	fairly broad	Thin
4	Radius	11/4 times of metacarpus length	Twice as long as metacarpus
5	Scapula	short & broad	Distinct neck
6	Spine	bent back & thickened	Straight and narrow
7	Sacrum	lateral borders thickened in the form of rolls	Lateral borders thin and sharp
8	Flesh	pale, red and fine in texture	Dark red & coarse in texture

Properties of meat and fat of various meat animals

Beef meat

- Meat is appealing and light red in young bulls
- Meat attains darker colouration in old bulls due to the role of testosterone

Veal meat

- Fat from some days old calves have jelly-like consistency and meat is pale and watery
- In baby calves both flesh and fat are of white colour which is acceptable
- As the age progresses, the fat of Jersey and Guernsey calves turn yellow

Mutton

- Mutton meat fibres are firm and fine and meat colour varies from light red to dark red
- Fat is white and firm with no odour

Goat

- Same in appearance as of mutton but classical goat odour of the meat
- Abundant kidney fat

Pork

- Pork is least firm meat
- Becomes white when cooked whereas in other species its becomes darker in colour
- Subcutaneous fat is more
- Pork fat is greasy, soft and white in colour

Horse

- Might be dark red or bluish in colour
- Odour is sweet and repulsive
- No marbling with fat

Chemical and biological differentiation of meat

Chemical tests

- Glucose content of horse flesh is quite higher than various other meat animals
- Detection of horse fat mixed with lard or beef or mutton fat by detecting 1-2% of linoleic acid in horse fat. Other animals fat do not contain more than 0.1% of linoleic acid
- Horse fat detection based on iodine value –
    - Iodine value of horse fat is 71-86, 38-46 in the ox, 35-46 in the sheep and 50-70 is pig fat (good lard: 66)
- Horse fat identification based on refractive indices: 53.5 for horse fat, less than 40 for ox fat and not above 51.9 in case of pig fat

Biological tests

The 3 important biological methods are:

1. **Precipitin test**
2. **Complement fixation test**

3. **ELISA test**
4. **Other tests— chemical procedures, microscopy, electrophoresis, agar gel diffusion, gas-liquid chromatography**

1. Precipitin test

- Test is particularly applicable to mince or sausage meat
- To test the presence of horse meat, horse blood serum is injected many times in rabbit
- The rabbit develops antibodies against the horse serum which precipitates the protein of horse and not the protein from other animals
- The horse meat detection test is performed in a test tube by mixing blood serum extracted from such repeatedly injected rabbits with the filtered extract obtained from the suspected meat sample
- Appearance of turbidity confirms the presence of horse meat in the meat sample

2. Complement fixation test (CFT)

- To detect the presence of horse meat in a meat sample, antibodies (Ab) are raised against the horse meat in some laboratory animal and the antibodies are separated out. Similarly, a blood component known as complement is recovered from guinea pig serum and sheep red cells or rabbit serum is used as indicator system
- In the suspected meat sample, specific antibodies raised against the horse meat are added
- If the meat sample contains the horse meat (target antigens- Ag), and Ag-Ab complex is formed
- Thereafter, complement is added which binds with the Ag-Ab complex.
- Then, sheep RBC is added and since, no free complement is available--- No haemolyis of the sheep RBC- Positive result--- meat contains horse meat
- In negative cases (no horse meat in the meat sample), no Ag-Ab complex will be formed and the added complement will be freely available and will lyse the added sheep RBC

3. Enzyme linked immunosorbent assay (ELISA) test

- ELISA in based on the inherent affinity of the antibodies to attach with the relevant antigens
- Specific antibodies (Ab) are raised in lab animals

- Suspected meat sample extract acting as antigen (Ag) is added to this specific Ab
- Ag-Ab complex is formed which is recognized by another Ab to which an enzyme catalyzing the reaction to produce colour is already attached
- The antibody which binds with the corresponding antigen forms a complex which is afterward recognized and bound by a second antibody containing an enzyme which catalyses the reaction to produce the colour.
- Colour is measured using spectrophotometer
- If the suspected meat sample contains horse meat and it is mixed with specific horse serum, the Ag-Ab reaction will proceed
- Even 3% horse meat addition could be detected by this method if the test is performed within 6 h

Meat composition and quality

- Protein is the most important constituent of muscle
- Muscle protein is made up of
  1. Myofibrillar protein- 2/3rd of total muscle protein (actin & myosin)
  2. Sarcoplasmic protein- Water soluble protein (myoglobin, haemoglobin, soluble glycolytic enzymes)
  3. Connective tissue protein—collagen, elastin & reticulin

Table 2.5: Muscle composition

S. No.	Constituents	% Net Weight
1	Water	75
2	Protein	19
3	Lipids (fats & oils)	2.5
4	Carbohydrates (glycogen)	1.2
5	Non-protein nitrogen	1.65
6	Minerals	0.65
7	Vitamins	minute quant.

1. Myofibrillar protein

- Provides muscle firmness
- Contribute to 2/3rd of total muscle protein
- Actin and myosin are the major myofibrillar proteins

2. Sarcoplasmic protein

- Proteins present in the cytoplasm of muscle cells
- Water soluble protein eg. haemoglobin blood pigments, myoglobin muscle pigment and soluble enzymes of glycolysis

3. Connective tissue protein

- Supporting mechanism of the body
- Consists of :
  - Collagen: water insoluble and converted to gelatin by heating
  - Elastin: tough yellow connective tissue
  - Reticulin: not converted to gelatin on heating

Lipids

- Mainly composed of triglycerides
- Other components of lipids are--- unsaturated and saturated fatty acids, phospholipids and different others fat soluble substances
- The horse flesh is high in intramuscular unsaturated fatty acids having iodine number of 75-80; cattle have a higher % than sheep, and pigs the lowest of these four species

Carbohydrate

- Muscle carbohydrate is mainly glycogen
- Glycogen occurs in liver also and high content in horse muscle and in fetus
- Glycogen is converted into lactic acid by anaerobic glycolysis
- Lactic acid production leads to fall of muscle pH from 7.2 to 5.5 (Ultimate pH)
- If the amount of glycogen at the time of slaughter is low, the lactic acid formation will be less and ultimate pH will be well above 5.5
- If the amount of glycogen at the time of slaughter is high, the lactic acid formation will be more and the muscle will reach ultimate pH of 5.5
- pH of the meat affects the water holding capacity (WHC) and the emulsifying capacity (EC) of the meat
- WHC is more when muscle pH is more

Non-protein nitrogen (NPN)

- NPN includes free amino acids, creatine, nucleotides, inosine monophosphate and carnosine
- Free amino acids and nucleotides give meat its flavour on cooking
- Some sugars (e.g. glucose) and lipids (certain lower fatty acids), nitrogen-containing compounds termed pyrazines and oxygen- and sulphur- containing compound also contribute to meat flavour

- Production of meat flavour is complex
- Factors affecting flavour of meat
    - More intense in fully grown animals than young animals
    - Veal has less flavour than bull meat
    - Breeds does not affect the flavour
    - Sex has major influence on meat flavour
    - Male has more pronounced flavour than female especially in pigs (boar-odour taint)
    - Fatness of animal is guarantee of good flavour and tenderness

Minerals

- Inorganic minerals constitute less than 1% of the muscle

Vitamins

- Meat contains a variety of vitamin B *e.g.* B1 (thiamine), B2 (riboflavin), niacin (nicotinic acid), B6 (pyridoxine), B12 (cyanocobalamin), pantothenic acid, biotin and folic acid
- Also vitamin A and C
- Pork contains 10 times higher thiamine (B1) than beef and lamb
- Beef has significantly higher folic acid than pork or lamb
- Liver- good source of vitamin B particularly thiamine
- Cooking reduces the quantity of vitamins present in meat

Other constituents

- Pigments such as myoglobin and haemoglobin
- Redness of meat-due to myoglobin content which is greatest in beef (0.30-1.0%), least in pork (0.06-0.40%) and poultry (0.02-0.18%)
- Myoglobin content is higher in male; old animal
- Heart and diaphragm muscles- rich in myoglobin

Meat quality

Factors affecting meat quality

1. Physical and chemical changes in meat
2. Rigor mortis

1. Physical and chemical changes

- Freshly dressed meat looks dark and sticky
- Water can be extracted from such meat with high force
- High electrical resistance
- After one or two days, it becomes lighter in colour and looks juicy and non-sticky when minced. About 30% water could be squeezed out
- Electrical resistance reduces to 20%
- The rates of these changes are affected by the surrounding temperature and the quantity of meat glycogen

2. Rigor mortis

- Rigor mortis is the most significant and the first PM changes in muscle after the slaughter
- It is characterized by contraction and stiffening of all the voluntary muscles accompanied by joints rigidity and muscle surfaces lose the transparency
- During rigor mortis, carcase temperature rises by 1.5 °C
- Rigor mortis first sets in the muscle that were best nourished and most active before slaughter
- Initiates from the head and neck and proceeds backward affecting heart first
- The highest intensity of rigor mortis is noticed in the left ventricle and hence, this heart cavity is normally free of blood on post mortem examination
- In normal animal, rigor mortis appears only 9-12 h after the death and reaches greatest stiffness at 20-24 h and thereafter, decreases
- The progress of rigor mortis is affected by
    - The surrounding temperature -- high temperature accelerates and low temperature retards rigor mortis
    - Health of the animal: in febrile animal—rigor mortis may be absent or scanty
    - Level of muscular activity just before slaughter – most important factor
- Rigor mortis commences when ATP (adenosine triphosphate) and glycogen reserve are used up

- Myosin (thick fibrils) and actin (thin fibrils) are joined by a bond resulting in the formation of actomyosin—stiffening of the joints and muscles
- In haunted animals, rigor mortis will set very quickly and also, it will pass off rapidly
- The longer the rigor mortis takes to appear, the longer is its duration
- Disappearance of rigor mortis is due to softening of the coagulated fibres by the autolytic fragmentation
- The low pH of the muscle retards microbial growth and the meat connective tissue are changes to gelatin on account of higher quantity of lactic acid thereby making the meat more tender on cooking
- The level of lactic acid rises to 10 folds at the maximum rigor mortis compared to living muscle *i.e.* 0.05% to 0.5 – 1% after 24 h of slaughter
- Immediately after slaughter, the flesh is neutral or slightly alkaline (pH 7 – 7.2) but it becomes acidic in 1.5 h
- In freshly slaughtered beef carcase, the pH will be 7.0 and it will reach pH of 5.5 (ultimate pH) in 18 h
- Absence of rigor mortis might be due to fatigue or fear or excitement prior to slaughter
- Too rapid development of rigor mortis might result in early putrefaction and greater drip loss

Debasement of food (adulteration and substitution)

- '*Wholesome*' is term which denotes as 'promoting or conducive to good health or well-being'
- The major chance of meat substitutions arises for high value meat with low value meat such as horse meat for beef, goat meat for lamb or *vice-versa* depending on the local preference, cat meat for rabbit and, earlier rabbit meat for chicken meat
- Other way of substitution is the inferior quality meat of large animal is sold as meat from superior quality steer and heifer meat
- Comminution increase the chance of meat adulteration as communited meat are most prone for adulteration
- Another way of substitution is the replacement of Grade A heifer and steer beef meat with that of *C. bovis*-infected meat after refrigeration
- Selling mutton but calling it 'lamb' is another way of substitution and deception

- Comminuted form of meat increases the probability of substitution and adulteration although meat cuts/parts may be substituted

Ingredients used for debasement of meat

- Various types of non-meat and meat based proteins are used to hide the actual meat level in the product on analysis. These ingrediets are termed as 'meat extenders' or 'meat substitutes'
- *Non-meat proteins* are vegetable proteins such as soya bean which can simulate meat appearance and texture
- *Animal-based proteins* are low value meat parts which are legally referred as meat such as dried blood, bone protein, pork rind, urea and blood plasma
    - Sometimes, a product may contain pork rind but does not contain pork flesh
    - *Cereal* is added in 'all-meat products' for its ability to absorb water and thus providing a drier look to the product similar to its natural form
    - Bones from animal are used to recover ossein or bone protein. Similar to pork rind, it is not a complete protein but is used in product after soaking it with four parts of water so as to substitute high value meat of equal weight
    - Urea-
        - Primarily used as fertiliser and animal feed additive
        - It does not have any nutritional value
        - Being water soluble, it is used in meat as a source of nitrogen and thereby increasing the value of protein on analysis
    - Normally, dried blood and plasma are used as ingredients for animal feed, pet food or fertiliser and only very little amount is consumed as black puddings
    - Blood and plasma are also added in meat products to enhance the meat content after rehydrating it with water
    - *Water-*
        - More water is used than required during curing in the form of cure solution
        - Additionally, polyphosphate is also used in the curing solution so that water loss during cooking can be kept at minimum
        - Further, tumbling or massaging of the cured meat is done to ensure maximum absorptiof curing solution

- Finally, the cured meat product such as cooked ham or shoulder will have more water in the form of curing solution cheating the consumer
- Although, consumers like moist ham but a legal limit should be drawn for the water content of cured meats

Effects of feeding on animal tissue

- Fat is far more significantly affected than muscle due to feeding specially fat colour and texture
- The fat is distinctly yellow cattle fed on grass than stall-fed cattle whose fat is white
- The yellow colour of fat is due to carotene, a pigment converted into vitamin A in animal body
- Carotene is abundantly present in fresh young grass, yellow maize, carrot, cotton cake *etc.*
- The three main constituents of mammalian fat are – olein, stearin and palmitin
- Palmitin acts as solvent of carotene and cattle and horse fat contains a large proportion of palmitin
- In Jersey and Guernsey breeds, fat is yellow—due to genetic factor favouring carotene deposition in fat
- Calves fed on milk- white fat
- The deep yellow colour of Iceland and Ireland sheep breeds fat – due to presence of recessive genetic factor which prevents oxidation of yellow pigment xanthophylls
- Pigs fed on swill- soft, unattractive and insipid taste fat- high level of unsaturated fatty acids- rapid rancidity
- Feeding pigs on fish meal- results in brownish yellow colour fat- known as brown fat disease

Abnormal odours and taints of meat

- Abnormal odour in meat is due to storage of other stuffs along with meat
- Acetone odour of meat- in cattle suffering from ketosis

The following factors contribute to the abnormal odours of meat

Feeding

- Fishy odour of pig meat due to excessive feeding of fish meal – due to presence of high fat content in the fish meal

- Fishy odour is avoided if the fish meal contains 3-7% fat
- Feeding turnip to cattle-abnormal odour
- Turnip odour of carcase- due to obstruction or rupture of oesophagus by turnip—unmarketable carcase
- In sheep, feeding turnip does not cause any bad odour
- In sheep, feeding fermenting beet causes rancid odour and soapy taste—due to beatine present in beet
- Feeding excess of sugar-beet tops to cattle- abnormal flavour of milk
- Feeding mixture of fish or soya bean meal and barley to lamb—fleece is damp and 'pig' odour
- Feeding of young garlic leaves to rabbits and cattle-phosphorus odour of meat

Absorption of odour by meat

- Drug administration before slaughter particularly in dairy cattle might results in abnormal meat odour and taste
- The odour of drug persists in the thickest part of the carcase
- Drugs which imparts off odour to meat are linseed oil, turpentine oil, carbolic acid, chloroform, asafoetida *etc.*
- During transportation with other food stuff, refrigerated meat adsorbs abnormal odour *e.g.* citrus odour adsorption by meat during sea voyage
- Odour is more readily adsorb by the fat
- Odour of oil and tar might occur similarly

Products of abnormal metabolism

- Sweet and repugnant odour in cattle flesh suffering from fever or close to parturition
- Due to milk fever—high amount of acetone in animal body—off odour

Sexual odour

- Male sexual odour is most apparent just after slaughter and in fatty tissue while the carcase is still hot
- With the chilling of carcase, the odour vanishes but on heating/cooking meat, it may come back
- Male sexual odour like 'Stale urine' odour in the boar meat or male goat
- Male sexual odour is due to male sex steroid androsterone
- Prevented by oestrogen treatment

- No sexual odour in ram or bull
- Boar odour persists in flesh for a considerable period of time after the animal is castrated
- Can be obviated if the boar pig is castrated before it is four months old
- 'Boar odour' is also detected in gilt due to oestrus
- 'Off flavour' or 'musty taint' encountered in poultry meat is due to chloroanisoles released by the microbes from the wood preservatives in certain type of wood shavings used in deep litter

Judgement of abnormal odour

- Meat of boars, castrated boars and cryptorchid pigs are of lower value because of boar odour
- Presence of sexual odour can be given as justification for seizure of meat as unfit for human food
- Boar odour is minimized if carcase is cooled immediately after dressing and disappears when it is minced and sausage is prepared
- Abnormal odour of meat associated with diseases or other conditions prejudicial to human health will render the carcase, offals and blood unfit for human consumption
- Meat must be rendered as unfit if boiling test reveals strong odour of drugs or disinfectants

Hot boning of meat

- Traditionally, meat is cut into different parts after about 18 h of cooling of carcase
- With the availability of deboning machineries nowadays at the slaughterhouses, it is possible to cut the carcase into primal cuts and then go for deboning or boning followed by vacuum packaging—this is called hot boning/ hot deboning
- Hot deboning should be done in room at 10 °C
- Hot deboning removes the muscles from the bones as an intact group of muscles
- Because of reduced cut surfaces in hot deboning, bacterial load is reduced
- Then, the deboned meat is vacuum packed and kept at 10 °C for 24 h followed by cooling at 0 to 1 °C and stored

Advantages of hot deboning/hot boning

- More effective cooling of meat—reduced refrigeration cost
- Higher meat yield
- Reduced amount of drip in vacuum pack
- Better colour uniformity
- Warm meat can be moulded

Disadvantages of hot deboning/hot boning

- Difficulty in synchronization of slaughter and deboning lines
- Hot meat less easy to cut and vacuum pack
- Fat difficult to trim when meat is hot
- Unconventional shape of the cuts
- High standard of hygiene is required

Vacuum packaging

Two basic systems of vacuum packaging have been developed

1. A low vacuum is drawn in a plastic film of copolymers with polyvinylidine chloride followed by use of metal clip to seal the pack and then heat-shrinking in hot water for 2 s – *e.g.* Cryovac bag
    - This is a two stage process where vacuum is created followed by shrinkage of the film in hot water
    - Drip is retained close to the meat
    - Sealing with metal clip results in few failures (1%)
    - Meat shelf-life is increased by 8-10 weeks
2. High vacuum is created inside a nylon/polyethene laminate film and then heat sealing the package without dipping in hot water
    - This a single stage process where vacuum creation and sealing in done at one location
    - Pouches cost less
    - Shelf-life of 4 weeks
    - Suitable for beef but not suitable for mutton or pork
        - As the high pH of the mutton or pork does not inhibits the growth of anaerobic bacteria
        - Punctures of films from mutton or pork bones are high
    - High failure rate because of meat juice preventing effective sealing and thus allowing air to re-enter

- Drip accumulates at one corner of the package making it unattractive
- A mixture of oxygen and carbon dioxide is added after vacuum creation and before sealing
- Oxygen maintains the attractive meat colour and CO_2 reduces bacterial growth

Requirements for vacuum packaging using the above two systems

- Initial bacterial load of the meat must be low
- Hygienic handing throughout the process
- Packages and boxes should be carefully handled- avoid stacking
- Storage temperature must be 0-2 °C
- Packaging films should not be punctured before use

Tenderization/conditioning/ageing/ripening of meat

Meat conditionings/ ripening

- When carcase is held at 0 to 3 °C (above freezing point of meat), all the changes that occur in meat at high temperature takes place but with slow rate.
- Enzyme action on fat leads to production of free fatty acids
- Proteolytic enzymes of meat bring about changes in meat protein
- All this is characterized by marked increase in the flavour, juiciness and tenderness of the meat which is known as condition of the meat
- Conditioning is brought about by the endogenous enzymatic action (autolysis/self-digestion) and not by bacteria
- Enzymatic action is completely inhibited at temperatures lower than freezing

Increase in tenderness of meat is caused by

1. Soluble meat protein obtained after passing off the rigor mortis during which meat protein is coagulated
2. Soluble meat collagen formation by the action of lactic acid on the meat collagen resulting in collagen softening and swelling
3. Proteolysis of meat protein by meat proteases such as cathepsin
    - Tenderness of meat is influenced by the age, breed, nutritional condition and amount of muscular exercise of the animal.
    - Amount of connective tissue present between muscle fibres also affects meat tenderness

- Tenderness of meat can be increased by hammering or muscle stretching—disintegration of muscle fibres; quick freezing before rigor mortis sets in ; by application of pretease enzymes like papain (papaya), bromelain (pineapple), ficin (fig) *etc.*

Tenderstretch method of hanging beef sides

- In this method, two sides of beef are hang by inserting a hook behind the Achilles tendon which leads to increased meat tenderness
- Hanging beef sides by inserting hook in the obturator foramen or 'pope's eye' located at aitch bone averts muscle shortening and thereby, prevents toughening of meat

Tenderization of meat by electrical stimulation

- New Zealand was first to use electrical stimulation (ES) to prevent cold shortening or toughening of meat occurring due to quick chilling of lamb carcase
- ES beef is as tender after 4 days as non-ES beef after 10 days of conditioning
- ES advances the rigor mortis by producing a pH of 6 in 2-3 h after slaughter
- Electrical pulses are passed through the carcase immediately after the slaughter causing contraction of muscle and thereby exhausting all the glycogen, ATP and creatine phosphate
- 700 V for beef carcase, 25 pulses per second for 1.5 min about 30 min after slaughter

Advantages of electrical stimulation (ES)

- Acceleration of tenderness and reduction in ageing time
- Avoidance of cold and thaw shortening
- Allow rapid chilling
- Better flavour and colour of meat
- Allow hot deboning
- Improves neck cleanliness of carcase

Pre-slaughter tenderizing

- Protease enzymes are used directly in the form of solution or powder to tenderize the meat cuts
- Proteases are obtained from different sources such as papain from papaya or pawpaw, bromelain from pineapple, ficin from fig, trypsin from pancrease *etc.*

- Introduction of protease enzymes in the food animals through vascular system just prior to slaughter will distribute the enzyme throughout the animal body- ProTen Process
- Papain solution (300 to 500 ml) is injected via jugular vein and animal is slaughtered within 10-15 min
- The enzyme is activated and tenderizes the meat when cooked (60-71 °C)
- Moisture pick –up must not exceed 3% of the tenderized product
- Disadvantages-
  - Tongue, liver and kidneys of the treated animal becomes over-tender when cooked
  - Chance of anaphylactic shock while injecting the protease

Mechanically recovered meat (MRM)

- Meat recovered from the bones of animals after deboning operation using machines and equipments is known as mechanically recovered meat
- Traditionally meat left adhered to bone after normal deboning process is recovered by use of knives- laborious, time-consuming and not able to recover all the meat adhered to bones
- 5% extra meat is recovered by mechanical method

Mechanical methods employ three ways to recover the meat adhered to bones

1. Wet extraction system
2. Screening system
3. Pressure system

1. Wet extraction system

- Bones are cooked or agitated in cold brine – loosening of meat from bones--- meat in solution called **bone stock**
- Useful for meat processors who utilizes the liquid bone stock for preparing meat products

2. Screening system

- Bones are crushed and then pressed against a screen which allows the soft tissue (meat) to pass through but not the hard bone pieces

3. Pressure system

- Powerful press are used to compress the uncrushed bones against a series of channels
- Meat is separated from a column of compressed bones

Composition of mechanically recovered meat (MRM)

- MRM composed of red meat, marrow, collagen, bone and fat
- Ca content should not be more than 0.25%
- Fluoride content of MRM does not affect the adults
- No health hazard associated with MRM and even beneficial to consumer on account of better nutrition to consumer
- Arsenic has not been found in MRM
- Mercury does not accumulate in bones – so no mercury in MRM
- Zinc content is same as that of manually recovered meat
- Chlorinated hydrocarbons and tetracycline residues are under the maximum tolerance level

3

Layout and Facilities Required for Slaughterhouse

Facilities required for buffalo, sheep and goat slaughterhouses

1. Lairage
2. Large enough slaughterhouse area-
   - Separate area for pig slaughtering
   - Slaughter line and area for operations such as singeing, depilation, scraping should be demarcated by a high wall of at least 3 m high or by an open space of 5 m width
3. For stomachs and intestines emptying and cleaning, there should be one dedicated room
4. Separate rooms for handling guts and tripe
5. Fat and hides, hooves and horns should be stored in separate rooms
6. Accommodation for sick or suspected animals; detained meat or seized meat
7. Chilling/refrigeration room
8. Room for veterinary services
9. Provisions for lavatories, wash basins, changing rooms, and showers
10. Facilities for veterinary inspection
11. Entry and exit of slaughterhouse should have control mechanism
12. Separation of clean and unclean area
13. Waterproof flooring of room where meat is processed
14. Provision for steam exhaustion and sufficient ventilation
15. Sufficient artificial or natural lighting
16. Adequate potable water supply
17. Adequate hot potable water supply
18. Effluent treatment plant (ETP)

19. Adequate equipments for cleaning and disinfection of hands and tools-availability of hot water at 82 °C.
20. Dressing equipments should be of stainless steel
21. Overhead rail system
22. Protection against pests
23. Instruments, tools and equipments should be non-corrodible and easily cleanable
24. Separate manure section
25. Place for vehicle cleaning & disinfection

Site selection for slaughterhouse

Facilities required at abattoir site are:

1. Enough water and electricity supply (water requirement is more than 1000 litres/tonne of dressed carcase weight for cattle, 3000 litres/tonne for sheep, 6000 litres/tonne for pigs).
2. Sewerage facility
3. Motor approachable road without any traffic congestion
4. For employees' convenience, it should be near to public transport
5. Located near to labour supply area
6. Area should be free from odours, dust, smoke, ash *etc.* generated from other nearby factories
7. Provision to demarcate 'clean' and 'dirty' areas and access to it
8. Located far from residential area to prevent odour and noise complaints
9. Near to livestock availability area
10. Ground should support solid foundations such as piling and should not be flood prone
11. Possibility of future expansion
12. Normally, city areas are to be avoided; rural and designated industrial area are selected

Water supply for slaughterhouse

- Adequate pressure of 20 psi
- Cold and hot water (not less than 82 °C) should be available
- Water storage tank should be large enough to contain one day's water requirement
- The required amount of water is as given below:

Table 3.1: Water requirement for different species of food animals in abattoir

Species	Water requirement (lts.)/day/animal
Buffalo/large animal	272
Sheep/goat	45
Pig	454

Note: 25% more than above requirement under pressure of 15 psi

Area size of the slaughterhouse

Approach road should be 6.10 m wide

Small abattoir – 1-2 acres of land (up to 30,000 units/year)

Medium abattoir– 2-4 acres of land (more than 50,000 units/year)

Large abattoir– 2-4 acres of land (more than 1,00,000 units/year)

1unit=1 bovine= 2 pigs= 3 claves= 5 sheep/goats

Lighting

- Whole slaughterhouse should have sufficient natural or artificial light
- Light should not alter the natural colours. Recommended light intensity at different locations should not be less than:
  - 540 lux at all inspection points at 1.5 m height
  - 220 lux in workrooms at 0.9 m height
  - 110 lux in other areas at 0.9 m height

Ventilation

- Adequate ventilation is a must to remove heat and steam and to avoid condensation and minimise microbial load in the environment
- It also removes odours, dust, *etc.* from the premise

Floor and wall finishes

Floor sloping in wet areas should have gradient 1:50 leading to drain. Floor area should have drains at the rate of 40 m2/drain. In the bleeding area, the floor gradient should be 1: 25. Drainage valleys should slope to drains in the valleys at a gradient of at least 1:25. The width of the valleys should be 60 cm.

- These should be such to facilitate easy cleaning-- all floors, wall coverings, finishes should be non-toxic and non-absorbent as well as the floors should be non-slippery
- Walls covering should be of light colour, non-absorbent, even, sturdy, hard and washable

Pest control

- Entry of rats, mice, birds, flies and cockroaches can pose dangerous threat as they also carry food pathogen
- To control rats: Use of narcotic baits (alphachloralose and pentobarbitone sodium baited on wheat with a sticker oil e.g. risella oil)
- Insecticide spray should be used

Buildings

The following buildings are considered necessary in a modern abattoir:

1. Lairage
2. Slaughter hall
3. Emergency slaughter hall
4. Refrigeration room
5. Detained meat room
6. Condemned meat room
7. Hide & skin storage room
8. Gut and tripe room
9. Offal room
10. Edible fat room
11. Cutting room
12. Inedible area
13. Dispatch area
14. Changing room
15. Manure bay
16. Vehicle washing area
17. Veterinary office
18. Laboratory

1. Lairage

- Area for resting of the animals awaiting slaughter after arrival at the slaughterhouse is called lairage
- Lairage space should be large enough to hold the number of cattle that can be slaughtered in three days and in case of sheep or goat or pig, it should hold two days'
- All animals should be handled gently and quietly
- Availability of water in lairage should be round the clock for animals
- If animals are to stay for more than 12 hours, they should be provided with fodder and feed

- Minimum resting period at the lairage should be 6 h for normal animals; 24 h for tired and agitated animals
- Maximum holding period at the lairage should not be more than 36 h
- Sick and suspected animals should be kept in isolation pen having solid walls and separate drainage
- Lairage gradient should be 2.5 cm for every 1.2 m
- Lairage pens for cattle can be made out of solid rendered block wall or tubular galvanised iron pipes having minimum height of 1.8 m
- Drive races (raceway) should be curved with solid side walls, non-slippery floor and sufficient light to facilitate forward movement of animals
- Drive races (raceways) leading to stunning area should be 'V' shape (called V-race)
- V-race dimensions can be 36 m length, 50 cm width at the floor and 80 cm width at the top
- Pen size should be 3-3.7 m wide

Table 3.2: Recommended space requirement for animals in slaughterhouses

S. No.	Type of animals	Space allowance
1.	Cattle (loose)	2.3–2.8 m^2/head
2.	Pigs (bacon and small porkers)	0.6 m^2/head
3.	Heavy pigs, calves and sheep	0.70 m^2/head

Cattle lairage

- Lairage pens should have 2.4 m wide gates
- Pens size of 7.6 m x 6 m should be used for 20-25 cattle
- Water required for cleaning lairage is 680 litres/ cattle

Sheep lairage

- Height of sheep pen should be 0.9 m having passages of 0.9 m width between the pens
- The rails of pen should not have gaps of more than 15 cm to prevent sheep head being struck
- Pen gates should be double-hinged as it facilitates easy passage of sheep/ pigs
- Provision for water troughs being kept at the height of 50 cm from the floor to control fouling

Pig lairage

- The horizontal rails around the pen should not have gaps of more than 15 cm to prevent pigs head being struck
- Water fogging devices should be available to cool the pigs as this reduces fighting and occurrence of PSE meat (pale, soft and exudative pork)

2. Slaughter hall

- Light intensity of 20 foot-candles (220 lux) throughout the hall
- Light intensity of 50 foot-candles (540 lux) throughout the inspection area

Stunning area

- 3 m wide area should be left between the stunning pen and opposite wall so as to allow enough space for falling of animals after stunning
- The animal may regain after stunning so vertical iron bars of height 1.2 m having 5 cm diameter should be erected at 40 cm gaps

Bleeding area

- The bleeding trough should be at least 1.5 m wide for buffalo and 1.1–1.2 m wide for sheep/goat
- Edible blood storage must be ensured at not more than 3 °C
- Bleeding time ---- 6–8 minutes
- For large animals: The height of the overhead bleeding and dressing rails should be about 4.9 and 3.4 m, respectively above the floor
- For sheep/goat and pig: The overhead bleeding and dressing rails should be 2.7 and 2.3 m high, respectively from the floor and in case of pigs, the bleeding rail should be 3.4 m high from the floor
- Collection of blood for edible purpose: *stainless steel hollow knife* which is connected with two pipes (one for anticoagulant (sodium citrate/ phosphate) supply and another for blood flow to collection pan) is used under hygienic condition
- The knife is kept inside the wound at the bleeding area by hand or with the help of a rotating endless screw

Overhead rail dressing (line dressing)

- Concept of line dressing of carcases evolved initially from Canada
- After stunning and bleeding, the carcase is carried along the overhead rails by gravity or motor operated mechanism

- Carcase keeps moving along the rail and during this movement, each steps of dressing is done by designated workers and thus, many workers are involved in dressing a single carcase
- Reduces the labour requirement
- Since various machines, tools and equipments such as brisket saw, hock cutters, hide puller, aitch bone cutter, *etc.* are used simultaneously for different dressing operations, the slaughter rates are higher
- 9 meat inspector and 1 veterinarian for initial and final inspection is required for slaughter rate of 60-75 large animals/h

Various types of overhead line dressing systems for large animals

Gravity rail system

- In this method, a spreader (gambrel) is used to suspend the carcases and single-wheel trolley or runner is also used
- Carcases are carried forward manually along the overhead rail by gravity to each working platforms where different steps of dressing are performed
- With this system, lower slaughter rates (10–40 large animal/h) can be achieved

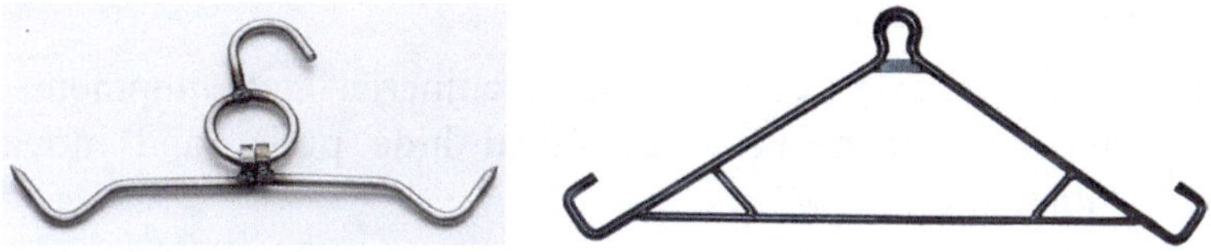

Fig. 3.1. Different types of gambrel

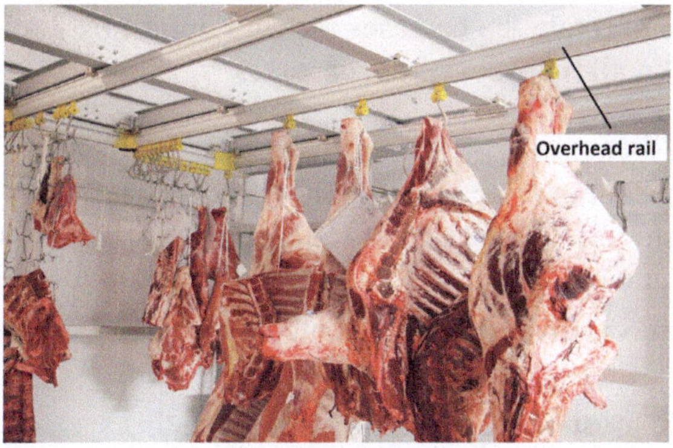

Fig. 3.2. Overhead gravity rail system

Advantages

- System is most compact and inexpensive than other systems
- Low probability of major fault and resultant loss of production as the system is most simple in design

Disadvantages

- Throughput is small
- Sufficient ceiling height is required so as to provide enough slope to the rail for easy movement of carcases with the help of gravity

Intermittent powered system

- Slaughter rate of 10–75 large animals/h can be achieved by this system
- Carcases suspended by gambrel (spreader) and trolley are pulled forward along the overhead rails by using motor and carcases are stopped at designated spots for dressing operations for variable time depending on the operation using pre-set timers

Continuous powered system

- The carcases move constantly without any stop along the overhead rails
- Higher slaughter rates (throughput) of 40–120 large animals/h is possible with system
- This system employs complicated machineries and equipments similar to 'Canpak' system like mechanical hide puller and movable-top inspection table
- Working platforms are equipped with adjustable height features to enable better working on carcases
- Provisions to rotate the carcases moving on rail by 360° so that worker can work on all the sides of the carcases

'Canpak' system

- Also a constant moving system where heavy beef trolleys or runners is used to hang the carcases from the overhead rail without using carcase spreader (gambrel)
- The system was invented and patented by Canada Packers Ltd., Toronto, Canada
- Nowadays, most of the slaughterhouses use this system
- Throughput of 50 to 150 large animals/h or more

Advantages of overhead line dressing systems

1. No chance for the workers to be idle because carcases keep on moving along the rail and worker has to perform the given task in a pre-set time
2. Safety is more with system compared to conventional slaughter systems
3. Dressing is hygienic since carcases are suspended on rail without touching the floor
4. This system eliminates the need for manual handling of heavy equipments such as trolleys, shackles and gambrels
5. Reduction in tedious work because of rotatable and height adjustable platforms and mechanised tools and equipments
6. More efficient, high throughput is achieved and increases the worth of carcase as well as of hide and offals due to better craftsmanship

Disadvantages of overhead line dressing systems

- Complicated machineries
- Requires regular industrial maintenance
- If there is any breakdowns in the line system, the whole dressing slaughtering and dressing operations have to be stopped
- Nature of the works are highly repetitive
- Meat inspection is difficult and not so efficient

Pig slaughter hall

- If pigs and other animals are slaughtered at the same time in any slaughterhouse, there must be a separate place for pig slaughter
- Nonetheless, such a separate place for pig slaughter is not required if pigs and other species of animals are slaughtered at different time
- But scalding, dehairing (scraping) and singeing must be performed at some designated place separated from slaughter line by a wall of minimum 3 m height or open space of minimum 5 m width

Scalding

- A scalding water temperature should be 60–62 °C
- Scalding time should be 6 min at 60 °C or 5 min at 61 °C for effective result.
- Generally, scalding at 60 °C for 5 min

Vertical scalding

- Consists of double-walled tunnel through which the pig carcases pass and during that passage, steam generated from tank kept below is driven over carcases causing scalding and finally steam is taken out by ventilator
- In the tunnel, the temperature is maintained at 61–64 °C
- This process takes 6 min
- After existing from the tunnel, scrapping and singeing is performed

Advantages of vertical scalding

- Reduces the microbial load of the meat, lungs are free from bacteria and decreases muscle degeneration
- Since the body temperature does not go rises above 41 °C, chance of PSE (pale, soft, exudative meat) is decreased
- Dehairing is improved and overall operational costs goes down

Scraping and singeing

- These are performed just after dehairing
- Singeing at 800–900 °C for 9–12 s. (in some case 1371-1537 °C)
- Singeing provides brown colour to skin, removes remaining hairs on skin and have preservative action

3. Emergency slaughter hall

- This is a small slaughter hall having lairage for accommodating four large animals fitted with overhead rail and hanging room

4. Refrigeration room

- To store meat at not more than 7 °C and offals at not more than 3 °C
- Hanging of carcases in such a manner so as to allow unhindered movement of chilled air around the carcases
- Spaces between the overhead rails in the refrigeration room for hanging the carcase sides of large animal, pigs and lambs should be 0.9, 0.7 and 0.5 m, respectively
- The spacing between carcase sides on overhead rails should be at least 0.3–0.4 m
- Freezing of large animal and pig carcases should be done at less than -7 and -15 °C, respectively and storage of beef and pig carcases should be performed at temperature less than -17 and -20 °C, respectively

5. Detained meat room

- Carcases which are held for additional examination are kept in this room
- All the carcase parts should be clearly identifiable till final decision is taken
- Light intensity should be at least 540 lux and it should not alter the original colour

6. Condemned meat room

- Adequate space, refrigeration and drainage should be available
- Lockable containers and weighing facility

7. Hide & skin store

- This place is used to stack and cool hides and skins.

8. Gut and tripe room

- Stomachs and intestines are separated and emptied in this room
- The ruminal contents being high in oxygen demand (COD > 100 000 mg/l) should not be released in the drainage system

9. Offal room

- Offals like heart, lungs, liver and kidneys should be kept in chill or freezing room
- Edible offals storage should be done at not more than 3 °C

10. Edible fat room

- Located close to gut room
- For storage of edible fat

11. Cutting room

- Its temperature should not be more than 12 °C during the cutting of carcases
- The meat and offals temperature should not exceed 7 and 3 °C, respectively in cutting room

12. Inedible area

- For storage of all inedible materials (unfit for human consumption)

13. Dispatch area

- This area must be far from dirty area
- Access restricted to vehicles only

14. Changing room

- For changing of the workers cloth while coming in or going out from the work

15. Manure bay

- Should be situated towards the dirty area of the abattoir close to the lairage

16. Vehicle washing area

- Should be located on the clean side of the plant
- Should be equipped with high pressure pipes, detergents and good drainage

17. Veterinary office

- Should be lockable room
- Should have hand washing and shower facility

18. Laboratory

- For preliminary diagnosis of the diseases
- Should be equipped to carry out trichinoscopic test

4

Transportation and Handling of Meat Animals and Its Effect on Meat Quality

Introduction: Relation between transportation and meat quality

One of the fundamental aims of animal production system is to ensure better quality meat. Apart from various animal husbandry practices that affect the meat quality, the transportation of meat animals from farm to slaughterhouse and their handling at lairage, affect the meat quality greatly. For better meat quality, the pH of the meat should fall from normal pH 7.0 - 7.2 in live animal to pH 5.5 (ultimate pH) after slaughter at the onset of rigor-mortis. The low muscle pH is required to inhibit the microbial growth and meat tenderization (cathepsins system is activated at low pH). The ultimate muscle pH is achieved through the accumulation of lactic acid which is produced as a result of anaerobic glycolysis of glycogen. After slaughter, as the oxygen supply to muscle ceases, ATP is generated through anaerobic glycolysis of glycogen and in this process lactic acid is produced. ATP is required to keep the muscle in relaxed stage. This anaerobic glycolysis carries on till the glycogen reserve is exhausted. So, higher the glycogen reserve at the time of slaughter, longer the length of time duration of anaerobic glycolysis and higher the quantity of lactic acid production and greater the reduction of muscle pH. Hence, livestock should be transported and handled before slaughter carefully because stress during transit and in lairage could severely deplete the glycogen reserve of livestock.

The following facts should be especially taken care by the farmers raising livestocks for meat

1. Housing arrangement and design

- Any flaws/deficiencies in design, layout, cubicle size and its design, drainage, water bowls, slats, air circulation, *etc.* should be rectified

2. Bedding

- Sufficient bedding is necessary
- It is paramount to start with a deep layer and later on keep adding bedding material at fixed intervals

- A concrete area is provided that should be regularly cleaned by scraping and this will decrease bedding necessities
- Slurry must be removed too often at fixed interval

3. Housing/stocking density

- Optimal housing density should be followed as higher or lower stocking densities results in dirty animals
- If the number of animals housed in slatted pen is less, the faeces will not get tramped through, will fail to fall down and will collect

4. Clipping

- Hairs around the bellies, briskets and flanks of the animals should to clipped to avoid the building up of matted manure on the hair

5. Management

- Better level of animal husbandry is required, particularly, when animals are housed for the first time
- Single animal that do not adopt to a specific housing system should be taken out
- It is better to encourage or train animals to rest in cubicle pens

6. Internal parasitism

- Deworming schedule duly approved by veterinarians should be followed to avert the possible occurrence of parasitic diseases in animals

7. Transport and abattoir lairages

- When animals are loaded at farm, they must be clean and this condition should be maintained during transportation so that the animals reach at the abattoir in clean condition

Clean livestock production

Contamination of cattle hides with manure

- Faecal contamination of hides, skins and fleeces poses many fold damage in the form of
  - Carrying pathogenic microbes such as *E. coli O157:H7, Salmonella, Campylobacter, Yersinia, Giardia, Listeria, etc.*
  - Contributes in the injury to hides/skins and finally to leather ('coarsened grain') by excoriating the uppermost strata of the skin and thus, revealing the sensory nerve endings resulting in pain and ultimately, compromising the animal welfare (Fig. 4.1)

- Chances of knife slips increase for the workers involved in dressing of carcases and thus, creating hazards for them
- Hides/skins contamination with faeces is creating problem for meat industry which is costing millions per year and the problem should be checked at mostly at farm, transportation and abattoir

Reasons of unclean livestocks

- The chief reason is the lack of bedding materials which is further intensified by many factors such as higher stocking densities, meagre ventilation resulting in water condensation, improper drainage, insufficient floor gradients and occasional cleaning of slurry
- In few cases, deficiencies comprising of improper cubicle size, incorrectly placed or overflowing water bowls or troughs, clogged slats because of non-removal of slurry and livestocks resting outside the cubicle or bedded area
- Presence of bigger livestocks and feeding of silage at farm further aggravate the problem
- Build-up of manure on the livestock around the long hairs found during the winter months contribute to dirty livestock

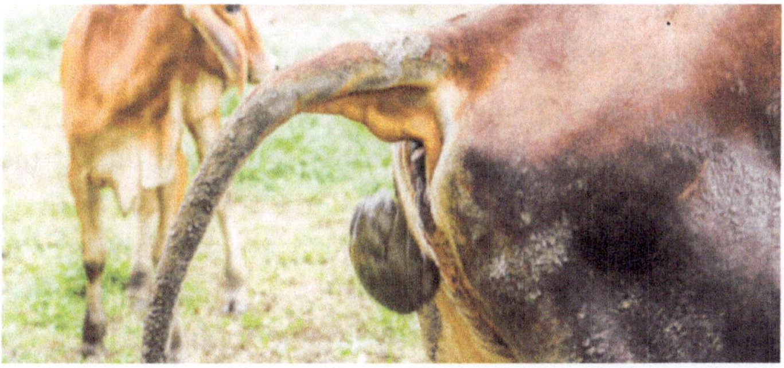

Fig. 4.1. Excoriation of the skin surface of large ruminant due to drying of dung on skin

Animal welfare at the farm level

- Animals welfare is regarded as the state of animals to deal with its environment
- Hence, animals welfare also contains degree of failure to deal with the environment which might result in disease or injury and also the easiness/difficulty to cope
- Therefore, animal health is connected with its welfare

An animal welfare during its stay at farm or in transportation or at market or at abattoir should be assessed in relations with the 'five freedoms':

1. Freedom from hunger and thirst

- This is ensured by easy availability of feed and water to sustain good health and wellbeing of animals

2. Freedom from discomfort

- This is made sure by giving proper housing and relaxing environment

3. Freedom from pain, injury and disease

- This is ensured by prevention or quick diagnosis of diseases and its treatment

4. Freedom to express normal behaviour

- This is made sure by adequate space, appropriate facilities and housing of animals of same species and same farm together

5. Freedom from fear and distress

- This is ensured by providing environment and treatment so that animals do not suffer any mental stress

Transportation of livestocks

- After raising healthy and clean meat animals at farm, it is required that the animals are kept in contamination-free conditions during the transport and at lairage
- It is of much significance that the animals do not suffer from stress, harm, weight loss and disease during the transport
- Due to above cited causes, it is advisable to rear animals as near to slaughterhouse as possible to avert journeys of long duration

Loading and unloading of meat animals

- Usually, the utmost stressful event of transportation is the loading and unloading of farm animals
- For pigs- a ramp with slope angled at 20–24° having cleats of 10–40 mm width and separated by 50–100 mm of distance
- For cattle- ramp used may have steps as in staircase or its floor may have cleats
- Ramp having stepped floors should be made up of concrete with 100 mm rises and 500 mm treads

- Wooden or concrete floors ramp should have cleats of dimensions 50 mm width and 50 mm high and spaced at 300 mm
- At most, a slope of 20° is suggested

The journey of livestock to slaughterhouse

Safeguard during transportation

- The workers involved in loading/unloading and transport of livestock should be well trained and experienced in such process and must not cause any undue pain, injury and fear to the livestock

Transport vehicles

- The transport vehicle employed should be designed, constructed, maintained and operated in such a way that it would prevent pain and injury and safeguard the livestock (Fig. 4.2)
- These are ensured by:
  - Easy cleaning and disinfection of vehicle
  - The facility of anti-slip floors
  - Sufficient lighting inside

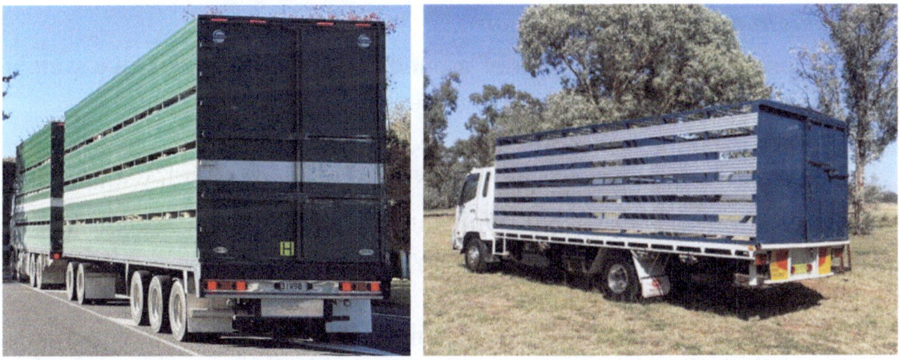

Fig. 4.2. Livestock transport trucks

Space requirement

- Adequate floor area and height must be ensured
- The allowed space and height should match the species and type of animals and the proposed trip

Duties of transporters

- The welfare of animals must not be negotiated and ensured by
  - Adequate harmonization of the various sections of the journey and
  - Taking care of the prevailing weather conditions

Feed, water and rest periods

- At adequate time gap, the animals should be provided with feed, water and rest which should be sufficient in both quality and quantity in relation with animal species, size, age *etc.*
- Usually, meat animals should not be conveyed for more than 8 h and if required beyond, further necessary provisions should be available in the vehicle
- Maximum duration of transportation for pig is 24 h
- Large ruminants, goat and sheep may be conveyed for 14 h before being offered minimum 1 h rest with water and feed (if required)
- Horses might be conveyed for a maximum of 24 h duration during which time, they are provided with water and feed (if needed) at each 8 h interval
- In case of poultry, if the journey duration is less than 12 h (24 h for chicks), there is no need of water and feed and for longer duration (more than 12 h for adult chicken and more than 24 h for chicks), adequate water and feed arrangement should be made

Loss of weight during transportation

- Pigs experience weight loss of around 2.2–5.4 kg of their live weight which is equivalent to 4–6% of body weight during 24 h journey
- In case of lambs transportation, carcase weight loss is almost 0.5 kg/animal/day if the journey duration exceeds more than 24 h without feed
- Rail transportation of large ruminants results in carcase weight loss to the tune of 1.48% up to the journey of 161 km and 2.1% during the journey of 402–482 km
- Weight loss in animal weight encountered during transit may partially (not entirely) be regained with proper and sufficient rest at lairage

Transport mortality

- Mortality during transit signifies extreme degree of stress in animals
- Any mortality rate more than 0 is not acceptable from the view point of animal welfare
- Deaths during transport is reported from several countries around the world but the occurrence is lower than 0.5% in all types of animals during transportation
- Death count during transport is more in hotter climate especially at more than 16 °C and if the vehicle is standing

- The death at 32 °C temperature during transit would be double than what observed at 16 °C

Lairage construction

- Livestock must be housed in lairage in such a way that inhibits any additional contamination of hides/skins, fleece and feet
- Lairage floor must be of concrete and non-slippery and sufficient gradient is provided towards the drain for easy cleaning (Fig. 4.3)
- Due to behavioural inquisitiveness, livestock movement is rapid if the raceways are curved instead of being straight and if the raceway has sharp corners, they will show significantly slow movement (Fig. 4.4 & 4.5)
- Lairage amenities should be inspected to prevent any death/injury due to some deficiencies
- In the lairage, any projections and sharp corners must be avoided
- Rails when used for partition of pens should be sufficiently spaced to prevent strucking of animals head

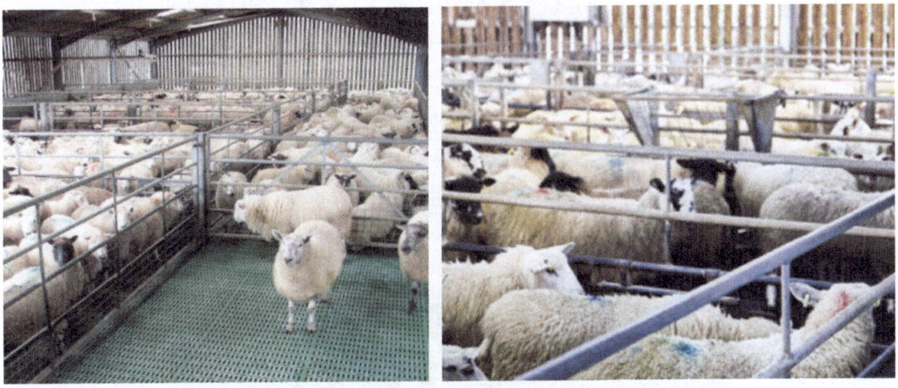

Fig. 4.3. Typical lairage pens for sheep

- In few countries, water jets are used to spray water on large animals before reaching the slaughtering area
- This provision is better in hotter climate where hair is small and livestock skin is thin
- Light spraying of pigs--prevents pigs fighting and also decreases the accumulation of contamination in the scalding tank
- The better quality meat obtained from pigs sprayed with water is because of body cooling and not due to lower level of stress

Facilities required to conduct ante-mortem examination efficiently in the lairage comprise

1. A race for identification of livestock having a crush gate for animals
2. Sufficient quantity of pens having enough light and provisions for identification or numbering of pens: a light intensity of 220 lux is must for ante-mortem examination
3. An isolation pen equipped with inspection facilities for specific livestock
4. Experienced and trained lairage worker for supporting the identification, movement and inspection of animals
5. Provision for veterinary office to complete the official documentation and records

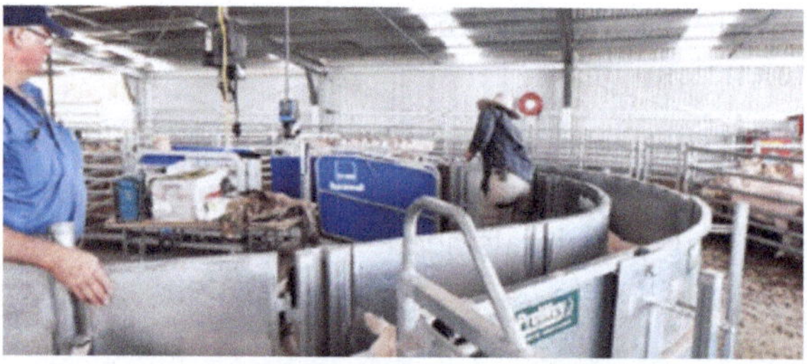

Fig. 4.4. Raceway is used to drive animals from lairage to slaughtering area

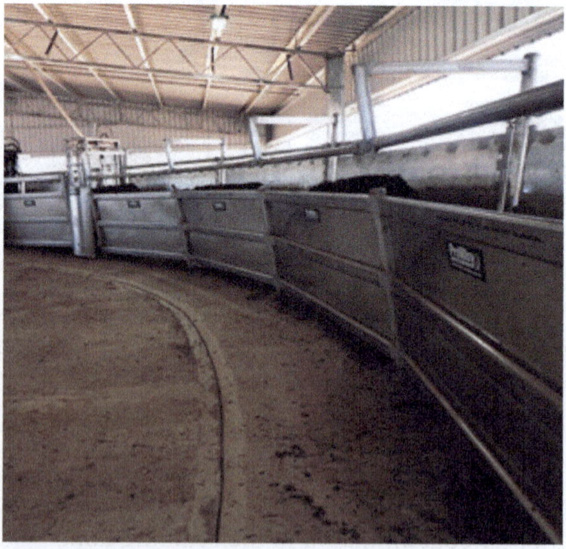

Fig. 4.5. Curved raceways are more useful to drive animals from the lairage to the slaughtering area (*Source:* https://proway.com.au/products/cattle-handling-products/cattle-race-options/v-race-34-sheeted-inside-fully-outside)

Management of livestock in the lairage

Driving livestock inside the lairage

- Pre-slaughter stress prevention is very essential just before slaughter because of
  - For economic causes of meat quality
  - For animal welfare aspects

  Hence, livestock should be handled gently with least use of force

Use of flight zone to drive animals from lairage to slaughtering area

- The livestock will start moving once the worker breaches the 'flight zone' of the animals so as to maintain its flight zone with respect to the worker
- The direction of movement is determined by the direction from which the worker enters the 'flight zone' of the animal
- If he enters from front side of the shoulder area, the animal will move backward and if he enter from toward the back side of the shoulder area, the animal will move forward
- If he approaches the animal from back side ('blind area'), the animal will not move either forward or backward

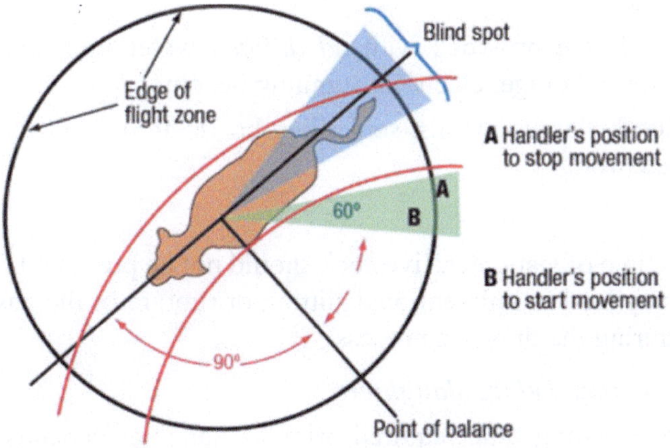

Fig. 4.6. Flight zone of animals
(*Source*: https://www.producer.com/livestock/sheep-smart-handlers/)

- Due to inherent behaviour of a sheep to follow the sheep moving ahead, a decoy or 'Judas' sheep which are trained sheep, are utilized inside the lairage to lead the whole flock
- Sheep are obviously terrified by the mere dog presence or its barking

- Pigs prefer to move side by side instead of moving one behind the other
- Hence, they move in a loose group of ideal size of 5 to 6 pigs
- Livestock, especially pigs are prone to stress if extreme or forceful noise is present
- Large ruminants are highly prone to high-frequency sound compared to humans

Social stress

- Keeping unfamiliar animals in the same lairage pen might result in fighting to institute a new social order and once this is established, the fighting stops
- Living with unfamiliar animals and subsequent fighting causes social stress
- This situation arises in lairage, in market place or during transportation of animals
- Violent animals, horned and polled animals and oestrus females should be housed separately

Watering

- Potable water should be available and accessible always for all the livestock
- If animals are provided with *ad libidum* water immediately prior to slaughter in lairage, electrical stunning becomes more effective
- Usually for large animals, self-filling bowls are more suitable than big concrete troughs

Fasting

- At the time of slaughter, livestock should not be presented full stomachs as it may lead to unintentional slitting or rupture of the gastrointestinal tract during the dressing process

Resting of livestock before slaughter

- The real resting time required prior to slaughter depends on the time duration to achieve normal physiological changes in the muscle and other factors
- These factors are the age, sex, species, class and condition, weather, means of transportation, distance of journey *etc.*
- Large ruminants should be given maximum rest of 4 h in lairage in effort to gain maximum carcase yield and optimum meat quality

- For pigs, 2–3 h a rest period is suggested
- Too much extended period of stay in lairage, besides increasing the chance of cross-contamination, makes the lairage dirty which is one of the most toughest cleaning task in abattoir
- Extending the period of lairage holding increases the accumulation of pathogens such as Salmonella particularly in pigs and calves as well as risk of cross-infection rises

Livestock handling prior to slaughter and its effect on meat quality

Stress related to meat animals

- Stress is non-specific response of an animal trying to repel or adjust to preserve homeostasis, *i.e.*, the tendency of the body to maintained the inner environment constant and equilibrium
- Two major reactions of an animal subjected to stress:

  I. The alarm or emergency reaction and

  II. The general adaptive syndrome

  Combinely, these reactions are called the fight-or-flight syndrome

I. The *alarm or emergency reaction*

- This reaction is shown by animals subjected to abrupt adverse stimuli and immediate in nature
- The stimuli result in enhanced sympathetic nervous activity resulting in higher activity of the involuntary muscles, the heart and the secretory glands
- All these leads to discharge of catecholamines, noradrenaline and adrenaline from the adrenal medulla gland which causes high blood pressure, increased heart rate and force of cardiac contraction, dilation of bronchi, stoppage of digestion, constriction of peripheral blood vessels and utilization of liver glycogen resulting in high blood sugar
- Glucagon, a peptide released by the α-cells of the islets of Langerhans in the pancreas, is more potent compared to adrenaline in the production of blood glucose by the mobilisation of liver glycogen

II. The general adaptive syndrome

- Contrary to alarm reaction which is in response to acute stress, the general adaptive syndrome is observed in response to stress of longer duration (chronic stress/ stress of longer duration)
- In chronic stress condition, adrenocorticotrophic hormone (ACTH) is released by the anterior pituitary gland and results in the production

of corticosteroids like cortisone and hydrocortisone (cortisol) which control the normal metabolism of carbohydrates, proteins and fats on a long-term basis

- Overall result is drop in carbohydrate metabolism and rise in protein metabolism leading to glycogen synthesis in liver from the amino acids
- Fat is transported from fat reserve to liver where fat is metabolized and ketone bodies are produced
- The conclusive result is elevated glucose and ketone bodies in blood
- General adaptation syndrome also causes hypertrophy of the adrenal gland and consequential decrease in its ascorbic acid and cholesterol stores, eosinophilia (decreased eosinophil count), lymphopenia (decreased lymphocyte count), polynucleosis (rise in polymorpho-nuclear leukocyte count) and higher vulnerability to disease

Pre-slaughter handling and meat quality

- Oxygen supply to the various muscles stops as the blood flow discontinues once the animal is slaughtered
- This leads to initiation of anaerobic respiration in the muscles as the typical aerobic respiration in the muscle ceases due to unavailability of oxygen
- During anaerobic respiration, anaerobic glycolysis takes place in which glycogen is degraded resulting in the production of energy (in the form of ATP) and lactic acid
- As the anaerobic glycolysis proceeds with time, more and more quantity of lactic acid is built up in the muscle causing normal muscle pH of 7.0–7.2 to fall to near 5.5 (**Ultimate pH**)
- This pH downfall usually takes 24–48 h in large ruminants, 12–24 h in goat/sheep and 4–8 h in pigs
- The energy production in the form of ATP (adenosine triphosphate) during anaerobic glycolysis is much lesser than aerobic form and so the quantity of ATP diminishes after slaughter
- Only 2 ATPs is produced in anaerobic respiration whereas 36 ATPs are produced in aerobic alternative from single glucose molecule
- ATP is essential to maintain the muscle in its relaxed condition
- So muscle will remain in relaxed stage after slaughter and rigor mortis will not occur as far as the ATP is supplied and it is utilized to maintain the relaxed state of muscle

- After slaughter, the diminishing ATP level reaches to a point where muscle cannot be in the relaxed state
- This situation causes the formation of irreversible bond between muscular components actin and myosin and thus actomyosin is formed
- Initiation of formation of actomyosin results in commencement of muscle contraction which is known as rigor mortis or otherwise called the carcase 'setting'
- Therefore, the time of commencement of rigor mortis is reliant on the quantity of ATP produced in muscles
- Hence, any outside factor that decreases the quantity of ATP production enhances the beginning of rigor mortis
- If the animal has depleted glycogen level inside the body due to poor nutrition or long distance transport resulting in exhaustion, the ATP production from anaerobic glycolysis after the slaughter cannot sustain for long time. This will cause early commencement of rigor mortis
- This is exemplified by the quick arrival of rigor mortis in carcase in fatigued large ruminants after the slaughter due to less amount of glycogen in the body resulting in less ATP production
- As discussed above, during anaerobic glycolysis, in addition to ATP, lactic acid is also produced
- If the glycogen reserve is less, there will be lower production of both ATP and lactic acid and hence, commencement of rigor mortis will be soon after slaughter and pH fall of the meat will be less (low amount of lactic acid production)
- Therefore, in such animals, the muscle pH will the high
- It is significant to note that the availability of ATP controls the beginning of rigor mortis and meat pH has nothing to do with the rigor mortis
- Pre-slaughter stress, hence, influences:

  i. Rate of onset of rigor mortis and

  ii. The rate and the extent of the fall in muscle pH
- Changes in these two above factors influences the meat appearance and quality
- The two frequently encountered examples of pre-slaughter stress are pale, soft, exudative (PSE) pork and dark, firm and dry (DFD) meat

Pale, soft, exudative (PSE) pork and dark, firm and dry (DFD) meat

- All muscle go through a drop in pH due to lactic acid production as a result of anaerobic glycolysis (ATP is produced) during the conversion of muscle to meat
- The classical pH fall in the pig meat would be pH drop to 6.5-6.7 from 7.0/7.2 at 37 °C after 45 min of slaughter
- On the other hand, in pigs which suffered from acute stress just prior to slaughter, the pH reduces to 6.0 or less than that just after 45 min of slaughter while the carcase is still hot
- This quick reduction of pH at high carcase temperature results in denaturation of meat proteins and thus, meat loses water holding capacity (WHC)
- The ante-mortem acute stresses include many factors at lairage such as rough handling of animals, high temperature, rough driving of the animals to slaughter area, mixing of unfamiliar animals, poor transportation condition *etc.*
- It is also suggested that the genes are related to occurrence of this condition with certain breed such as Danish Landrace, Pietrain and Poland China
- PSE meat condition is said to arise when the pH of meat falls to less than 6 within 45 min post-slaughter while the carcase is still hot
- Contrary to PSE, DFD (also called dark cutting beef) occurs when the ultimate pH reached 12 – 48 h after the slaughter of animal is more than/ equal to 6 (≥ 6).
- PSE and DFD conditions have major effect on fresh and processed meat
- Fresh PSE has more chance of it being rejected by consumers because of its appearance and its hampered physicochemical properties make the product preparation out of it a tough challenge for meat processors

Causes of PSE and DFD

- Stress during ante-mortem is the foremost cause of PSE and DFD conditions of meat
- Animals experiencing acute stress or short term stress immediately prior to slaughter results in PSE meat
- Fights between animals, application of electrical goads, overcrowding in lairage, beating animals just prior to slaughter are some examples of acute/short term stress

- Sudden fall in pH within short period of time is due to production of good quantity of lactic acid from the anaerobic glycolysis of glycogen after the slaughter
- Certain breeds are more prone- Danish Landrace, Pietrain and Poland China– endocrinological imbalances due to selective breeding- prone to post-mortem glycolysis

Factors contributing to PSE meat condition

- Rough ante-mortem handling
- Physiological differences between breeds and individual muscles
- Inefficient slaughter technique
- Inefficient handling of carcase

PSE (Pale, soft and exudative) conditions of meat (Watery pork)

- This meat condition arises because of rapid fall of muscle pH after slaughter while carcase is still hot (Fig. 4.7)
- The quick fall of pH is due to high lactic acid production resulting from higher rate of anaerobic glycolysis
- The low pH combined with high carcase temperature leads to denaturation of muscle protein which causes decreased water holding capacity (WHC) of muscle
- Poor WHC forces myofibrillar proteins (the myofilament lattice) to release fluid into the extracellular space
- Cutting of such meat causes release of exudates due to low WHC
- The higher amount of sarcoplasmic fluid than in myofibrils increases the differences in refractive indices of sarcoplasm and myofibrils
- Light scattering would be more if the differences in refractive indices is more resulting in the paler meat appearance
- PSE meat is serious issue if sold fresh
- Drip loss of up to 10% of weight; meat becomes tougher when cooked
- Takes more brine than normal pork during curing but curing is satisfactory
- Exudative ham might lose 2.2% or more weight than normal ham
- Large pig meat processors do not consider PSE as serious because they mix PSE and normal meat and so, the difference becomes less evident

Acute pre-slaughter stress in pigs

↓

Rate of anaerobic glycolysis is more

↓

Rapid production of lactic acid

↓

Quick fall of muscle pH (from 7/7.2 to ≤ 6) within 45 min of slaughter while carcase is hot

↓

Low muscle pH & high carcase temperature

↓

Muscle protein denaturation

↓

Reduced water holding capacity (WHC) of muscle

↓

Myofibrillar protein releases fluid into the extracellular space- High drip loss--watery appearance of meat & soft to touch

↓

Increased differences in refractive indices of the sarcoplasm and myofibrils

↓

Increased light scattering--- meat appears pale

Fig. 4.7. Flow-chart explaining the pale, soft and exudative (PSE) meat condition

Procedures to reduce incidence of DFD & PSE meat conditions

- Gentle and quiet handling of animals at farm and abattoir
- Loading and unloading ramp at farm and abattoir
- Original social order should be maintained at lairage
- Availability of *ad libidum* water and food when necessary
- Aggressive and oestrus animal should be isolated
- Overhear fine spray of water in lairage
- Use of sticks and electrical goads should be avoided
- Feeding of sugar in liquid form in lairage- replenishes glycogen
- Careful breed selection for slaughter
- Selection based on halothane sensitivity test

Porcine stress syndrome (PSS) (fatal syncope, shock heart failure syndrome)

- PSE is closely related to porcine stress syndrome and malignant hyperthermia
- PSS is characterized by sudden death preceded by elevated temperature, skin blanching, erythema, and dyspnoea in fat pig which have undergone stress

- PM examination of such carcass would reveal diffuse and severe degeneration of skeletal muscle with excess pericardial fluid
- Pietrain and Landrace are prone for PSS
- Pigs showing sensitivity to Halothane test are prone to PSS and consequently to PSE meat
- So, to detect the pigs susceptible to PSS, Halothane Sensitivity Test is performed

Halothane Sensitivity Test

- Halothane sensitivity is due to single recessive gene
- Pigs aged 3-11 weeks are given halothane anaesthesia and their reaction is termed positive if extreme rigidity of hind limbs are observed
- Male breeding pigs are selected based on this test and thus only pigs showing negative reaction for this test are selected for breeding

Disadvantage of halothane sensitivity test

- High mortality rates among the positive reactors

DFD (Dark, firm and dry) condition of meat

- DFD meat is encountered when animal is subjected to chronic or long duration stress prior to slaughter (Fig. 4.9)
- Poor feeding at farm, lengthy transport of animals, unavailability of feed for long period, congestion in lairage for longer period are some of the instances of chronic or long duration stress prior to slaughter
- Under these situations, there is reduction in glycogen reserve and hence the quantity of lactic production from anaerobic glycolysis is low thereby, the ultimate pH of the muscle remains high
- Such a condition leads to dark, farm and dry meat
- The low level of lactic acid causes very little muscle protein denaturation and WHC remains high and the sarcoplasmic fluid is withheld inside the myofibrils
- So, there is no loss of exudate on meat cutting and from drip loss. This makes meat appear dry
- Dissimilarities in refractive indices of the myofibrils and sarcoplasm is less as the water movement from sarcoplasm to extracellular spaces is little
- Hence, there is little light scattering and muscle absorbs more light making it appear dark

- Due to the lack of water movement from sarcoplasm to extracellular spaces, the myofibrils are densely packed limiting the oxygen diffusion inside the muscle
- Little amount oxygen penetrating deep inside the muscle is quickly utilised by high cytochrome activity stimulated by the high pH—further aids in darker colour of muscle
- Therefore, a slim layer of red oxygenated myoglobin (MbO2) is formed at the meat surface which is bright and inside the muscle, due to lack of oxygen, reduced myoglobin (Mb) is formed which appears purple colour
- This purple colour is visible from outside which provides unpleasant colour to DFD meat
- DFD meat is fit for human consumption
- But less desirable colour and lower keeping quality
- Not liked by meat retailers

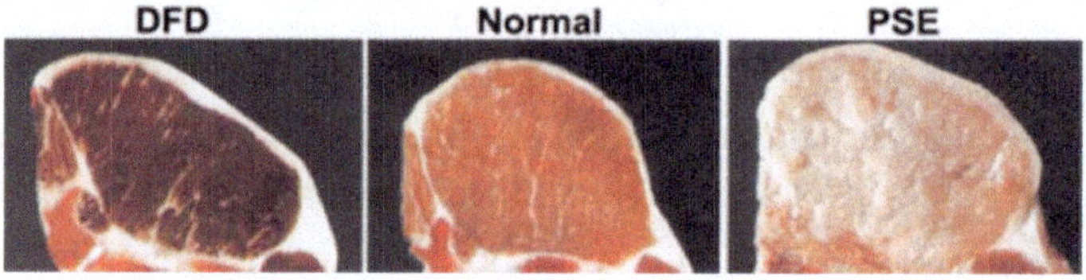

Fig. 4.8. Visual differences between DFD, normal and PSE meats (*Source:* FAO)

Chronic pre-slaughter stress in large ruminants

↓

Low glycogen reserve

↓

Less production of lactic acid

↓

Muscle pH remains high (≥ 6) even 12-48 h after death

High muscle pH

↓

Very little muscle protein denaturation

↓

High water holding capacity (WHC) of muscle

↓

No fluid release from myofibrils into the extracellular space-Dry & firm meat surface

↓

Reduced differences in refractive indices of the sarcoplasm and myofibrils

↓

Low light scattering/ light is absorbed--- meat appears dark

Fig. 4.9. Flow-chart explaining the dry, firm and dark (DFD) meat condition

Table 4.1: Differences between PSE and DFD meats

S. No.	PSE Meat	DFD Meat
1	Acute and short duration stress just before slaughter	Chronic and long-lasting stress before slaughter
2	Faster glycolysis rate after slaughter results in low pH (≤ 6) within 45 min when the carcass is hot	Reduced glycogen reserve prior to slaughter leads to high ultimate pH (≥ 6) even after 12-24 h of death
3	Pale, soft and exudative meat	Dark, firm and dark meat
4	Glycogen level is normal and fast muscle acidification due to rapid post-mortem glycolysis	Reduced glycogen reserve and hence, less acidification (high pH)makes meat more prone to spoilage
5	Muscle protein gets denatured	No denaturation of muscle protein
6	Large extracellular space in muscle fibres	Small extracellular space in muscle fibres
7	Reduced water holding capacity (WHC) of meat	High WHC of meat
8	Meat scatters more light	Meat scatters less light and absorbs more light
9	Myoglobulin absorbs less green light	O_2 is consumed by high cytochrome action
10	Meat appears less red	Meat appears dark

Steps to prevent occurrences of PSE and DFD in meat

1. Avoidance of pre-mortem stress in animals
2. Halothane test
3. Pre-slaughter feeding of sugars

1. Avoidance of stress

- Animal should not experience stress while they are at farm, during loading and unloading from vehicles, long time feed and water unavailability while in transit, keeping unfamiliar animal groups together at lairage, hot environment, noisy surroundings *etc.*

2. Halothane test

- The halothane gene was inherited from the Piétrain breed
- This breed was selected for breeding to enhance the muscle growth since it normally carries the double muscle gene
- Thus, pig lines obtained from Piétrain commonly carries double recessive halothane gene and such pigs may die due to stress or tend to produce PSE meat if survives the stress
- Halothane sensitivity is caused by single recessive gene

- Prospective breeding pigs are exposed to halothane gas because pigs which are 10 weeks old and carrier/ double recessive for this gene will show rigidity of hind limb– Positive case PSE prone
- Exposing all potential breeding pigs to the anaesthetic gas halothane because it was found that if 10-week-old pigs which were carrier/ double recessive for this gene were exposed to this gas, hind limbs would become rigid
- Pigs which does not possess halothane gene maintained a relaxed position
- Lately, a gene probe has been devised which is low-cost and more welfare acceptable

3. Feeding of sugars before slaughter

- To replenish the glycogen reserve of the animal muscle so that required pH fall is achieved following slaughter due to adequate lactic acid production, it is essential
  - To reduce stress, fear, tiredness, excitement or undue exertion of the animal
  - To give enough rest period to animals in lairage so as to regain the glycogen level in muscle
  - Additional measure is to provide the animals in lairage with readily digestible source of sugar so that glycogen level is restored quickly
- Therefore, molasses are fed to animals in lairage through drinking water
- Sugar feeding quickly replenishes the glycogen reserve of the muscles and liver which acts as energy source enabling the muscles to achieve the low pH due to adequate lactic acid production

Traumatic injury of the meat animals

- Bruising is defined as traumatic injury without penetration of the skin where blood vessels are damaged to such an extent that there is extravasation into the surrounding tissues.
- It is important to determine the time of bruises so that it could be ascertained whether the bruises were caused in the farm or during transportation or in the lairage
- Thus, determining the timing of bruises will help the manager to rectify the problem at farm or during transportation or stay in the lairage
- Large ruminants bruising mostly occurs at the loin and hip area and the shoulder

- In sheep, many of the bruises are due to rough handling, resulting either from animals being lifted by the wool or grabbed by the legs during sorting, weighing and loading on the farm, during unloading or while being handled prior to being stunned
- Fasting increases bruising and chronic stress makes animals more susceptible to it

Methods of dating of bruises

1. Bilirubin test
2. Physical appearance method
3. Electrical conductivity method
4. Histological methods

1. Bilirubin test

- Based on the formation of bilirubin from haemoglobin in the area of the bruise
- A sample of bruised meat is soaked in Fouchet's reagent (trichloracetic acid and ferric chloride)
- Bruises up to
  - 50 hours old---no reaction;
  - 60–72 hours old---turn the solution light blue
  - 4–5 days old--- dark-green reaction

2. Physical appearance method

Table 4.2: Approximate ageing of bruises by physical appearance

Time period	Appearance of bruise
0–10 hours old	Red and haemorrhagic
Approximately 24 hours old	Dark coloured
24–38 hours old	Watery consistency
Over 3 days	Rusty orange colour (bilirubin) and soapy to the touch

3. Electrical conductivity method

- By measuring the electrical conductivity of the tissue, which increases up to a maximum at 40 h

5

Ante-mortem Examination of Meat Animals

Introduction

- Meat inspection involves proper veterinary examination of live food animals prior to slaughter (called ante-mortem examination), inspection of carcases and offals and pathological examinations where deemed fit
- Full ante-mortem inspection represents 50% of meat inspection
- Ante-mortem inspection is particularly useful for detecting scheduled or infectious diseases which are communicable to man e.g. anthrax, rabies and glanders
- Diseases where animals show nervous symptoms like tetanus, tuberculous meningitis, sturdy in sheep, lysteriosis, rabies, cysticosis *etc.* and where skin lesions are manifested such as food and mouth disease, swine fever *etc.* are easily detected during ante-mortem inspection which are difficult to be detected in post-mortem inspection
- Animals must undergo veterinary ante-mortem inspection on the day of their arrival at the slaughterhouse or before the beginning of daily slaughtering

The inspection must determine

1. Whether the animals are suffering from a disease which is communicable to man and to animals or whether they show symptoms
2. Whether they show symptoms of disease or of a disorder of their general condition which is likely to make their meat unfit for human consumption-- any medicine/substances
3. Whether they are tired, agitated or injured
4. Whether they are sufficiently clean to enter the normal slaughter protocol
   - For public health purposes, the veterinarian must separate normal animals from those which may be suffering from a potentially zoonotic disease or present a hygiene risk to the slaughter hall environment owing to the soiled condition of their hide/fleece

Important points for ante-mortem inspection

i. All animals for slaughter must undergo ante-mortem examination within 24 h of arrival at the slaughterhouse

ii. Inspection should be repeated if more than 24 h have passed since first examination

iii. Adequate lighting for inspection

iv. Ante-mortem inspection should determine

   a) If the disease is transferable from meat to human or to animals if the animal is showing some disease symptoms

   b) If the disease or disorder shown by the animal is likely to render the meat unfit for edible purpose

v. Animals shall not be slaughtered for human consumption:

   a) If they meet above two criteria

   b) If they are not rested adequately— 24 h should be given for stressed and fatigued animal

vi. Animals meeting the above two criteria (iv. a & b), must be kept in isolation pen

Ante-mortem inspection facility

- *Facility to identify the live animals*
  - Ear tags are used
  - Electronic identification – subcutaneously implanted transponders
- Lairage pen should be well lit
- Isolation pens
- Assistant staff for handling of animals

Process of ante-mortem examination in the slaughter premises

The *animal health* aspect entails the veterinarian to recognise *notifiable disease* for example foot and mouth disease or swine fever (serious epizootic diseases) which could be identified first at slaughterhouse similar to foot and mouth outbreak incidence in the UK in the year 2001

The veterinarian may take one of the five decisions given below after the ante-mortem inspection:

1. Animals may go ahead for usual slaughter
2. Animals must not go inside the abattoir or must be condemned ante-mortem.

- Dead, moribund, emaciated or markedly dirty animals and animals exhibiting symptoms of a septicaemia or other conditions leading to meat being unfit for edible purpose

3. Animals should be slaughtered but may require a special thorough post-mortem inspection, or may require to be slaughtered in a designated place or at a separate time from other food animals
    - Animals having localised infection or generalised condition
    - Animals fed with illegal drugs for enhancing the growth rate or having residues of medicinal drugs/ingredients
4. Animal slaughter allowed with some conditions- *e.g.* dirty flock at a slow line speed
5. Slaughter may be delayed- for extremely exhausted or agitated animals or those needing treatment

The decision taken at the ante-mortem can be summarized as follows

i. Approval for slaughter
ii. Condemnation
iii. Slaughter allowed under special precaution
iv. Delayed slaughter
v. Casualty slaughter

Practical way of ante-mortem inspection process

- In lairage, animals should be examined both while relaxing and walking
- Animal should be inspected from both sides
- Carried out while the animals are being unloaded
- The overall activities of the animals, fatigue or excited state, general health condition, signs of any disease, nutritional status and any deviation from normality should be looked and noted down
- Animals exhibiting disease signs and febrile condition must not be slaughtered for edible use
- Segregation of diseased and suspicious animals, oestrus female, aggressive animals, horned and polled animals
- Crowding of animals in vehicles and its cleanliness is noted
- Birds suspected of communicable (like ornithosis) and notifiable diseases (like Newcastle disease) should be looked carefully for the clinical symptoms

- Animals suffering from fever and systemic problems should not be allowed for slaughter and retained for treatment
- Suspected animal must be specially marked and carried along with veterinary report to the meat inspector as well as the lairage staff and operators working in slaughter line *e.g.* in case of ringworm and contagious pustular dermatitis
- Special attention must be paid to recumbent animals—either it is instantly condemned or allowed for instant slaughter or withheld for additional inspection
- Suspected animals are those animals who are likely to be suffering from disease or suffering with disorders that shall lead to carcase condemnation on PM examination such as in cases of downers cow syndrome, leptospirosis, anasarca, swine erysipelas, vesicular stomatitis, TB reactors, anaplasmosis *etc*.
- Diseases or conditions where carcases are condemned include food animals in comatose or semi-comatose condition, animals displaying signs of certain toxic, metabolic, nervous or circulatory disorders—anaplasmosis, listeriosis, ketosis, leptospirosis, tetanus, grass tetany, azoturia, scrapie, glanders (farcy), swine fever, anthrax *etc.*
- Records of ante-mortem results are stored and should be presented during post-mortem examination so that those results could guide at the PM examination

Emergency slaughter of food animals

- Animals in acute pain (due to accidents *etc.*) are allowed to be slaughtered at the animal farm to alleviate the suffering of the animal and then carcase is transported to slaughterhouse along with veterinary certificate and other history related to animal
- Contrary to the normal regulation that only live livestock could enter and is slaughtered at the abattoir, emergency slaughter allows animals to be slaughtered at farm and then brought at the abattoir for human consumption
- Emergency slaughtered animal meat can be declared fit for human only if the animal was healthy before meeting with an accident and it suffered from acute pain which prevented its live transportation to slaughterhouse considering the animal welfare
- Emergency signifies that animal was suffering from acute pain due to some reasons such as accidents, limbs fractures, life-threatening injuries, profuse bleeding and hence, slaughtered at the animal farm

The judgement at the farm in emergency slaughter

- If in the opinion of the livestock owner (farmer), the animal was healthy and fit for consumption, he would call private veterinary doctor for his advice
- The veterinary doctor has to take one of the following three decisions:
  1. The animal is suitable for live transportation to the slaughterhouse as well as for human consumption and is sent along with full feeding chain history
  2. The animal is allowed to be slaughtered at the farm and carcase taken to the slaughterhouse along with full feeding chain history and veterinary doctor certification to this effect
  3. The animal is allowed to be slaughtered but must be condemned as animal byproduct

Categories of emergency slaughter animals that may arrive at slaughterhouse

I. The animal reaching alive but in comatose state

- Total condemnation of carcase

II. The animal reaching dead and not dressed

- Such carcase will show engorged veins and capillaries because of lack of bleeding
- High blood content of lungs, liver and kidneys
- When carcase is opened, greenish hue is observed on abdominal wall and kidney fat
- Liver surface- yellow to greenish hue due to imbibition of bile
- Unloading of such animals at slaughterhouse premise should not be allowed
- Rule out anthrax
- Total condemnation of carcase – due to imperfect bleeding
- Carcases of dead animals are not wholesome, prone for rapid deterioration and should be sent to rendering plant

III. The animal may arrive in the form of a dressed carcase

- Great difficulty in judging such carcases
- Head should be observed for stunning signs—this will indicate bleeding after stunning

- In dead eviscerated animal, carcase surface has whiter appearance if hide removal is delayed by few hours
- Decision will depend on bleeding status, absence of disease, PM examination of organs and lymph nodes

The acceptance decision at the slaughterhouse in the event of emergency slaughter is based on

- Whether the feed chain history and veterinarian testimony are brought to the slaughter establishment or not
- The veterinary doctor are required to declare that the carcase could be processed for human consumption
- A comprehensive post-mortem examination must be done
- Animal tissues samples should be preserved for diagnosis of suspected diseases especially drug residues

Casualty slaughter

Casualty slaughter is the slaughter of animal at the slaughterhouse after the animal has been certified fit for transportation from farm to slaughterhouse. These animals may be affected with more chronic conditions like mastitis or chronic arthritis, lameness etc.

6

Post-mortem Examination of Animal Carcases & Offals

Post-mortem (PM) examination

The core objective of post-mortem examination is to identify and eradicate defects and contaminations and thus, confirming that only meat suitable for ingestion are allowed to be passed

Facilities for post-mortem inspection

- Normal infrastructure amenities which delivers comfortable working environment and assist in presenting the carcases and its offals for PM examination
- Every inspection place on the dressing over-head line must have lights of -- 540 lux (50 foot-candle) intensity light which does not alter the normal colours
- Adequate facility for sanitising the hands, equipments and aprons should be provided
- To sterilise the knives, cleavers and saws–a water bath operating at 82 °C
- Head, viscera and carcase are the three major inspection parts
- On moving rails, viscera from a particular animal should move little ahead of its carcase so that any abnormality in viscera could be conveyed to the carcase examiner well in time
- For precise recognition of carcases and its correlated viscera from an animal, the lines conveying the carcases and viscera should move in synchronized way
- When a carcase is declared unfit for human consumption, all its the related parts such as head, viscera, blood and hide must be collected and disposed off
- Every inspection point must have a easily accessible overhead rail line stop button

- If there is any incidence of contamination or loss of synchronisation between the lines, the lines must be stopped instantly

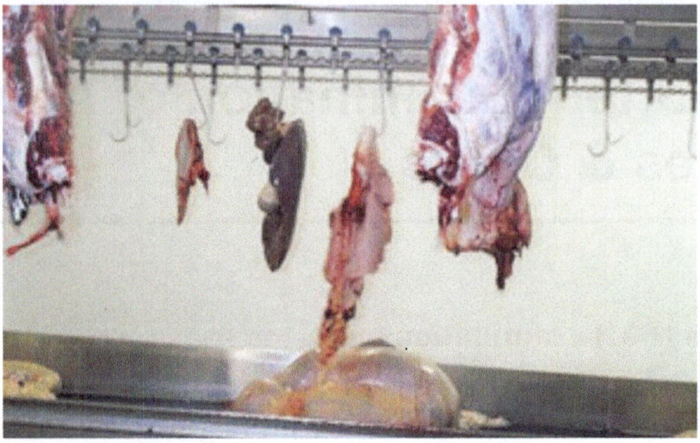

Fig. 6.1. Synchronized movements of carcase and its related viscera. Note that the viscera is moving little ahead of its associated carcase (Reproduced from Harold Moore)

Carcase identification and traceability

- The identification system used on animals when it was alive and at farm, should be left as such on the carcase
- If for hygienic reason, the tags from the live animals are removed, there must be a robust system of identification of the carcases
- Plastic or metal clips that are frequently applied on carcases for identification must be removed before the carcases enter into deboning room
- The practice of retaining the tags on large animals as its carcases moves through the slaughter line has clearly some advantages *vis-a-vis* few drawbacks regarding carcase hygiene
- The use of *transponders* implanted in the ear which can be read at the inspection and grading/weighing points
- Transponders are utilized for carcase identification by implanting it in the animal ear and it can be read at various points such as inspection, grading, weighing *etc.*
- Additionally, marking dyes are put using metal/polypropylene stamps for carcase identification
- The carcase identification system should be simple, easy to apply, read without any difficulty, economical, harmless, non-rusting and must be compatible with modern electronic gadgets for dada handling

Guidelines on the labelling of carcase meat and prime cuts

1. Labelling, writing and stamping is done only if it deems necessary
2. Labelling should be always done at a fixed point of the carcase/primal cuts to help in easy reading and removal
3. Label should not be fixed to an area which has more chance be used for preparation of products *e.g.* flank and brisket
4. Once the objectives of labels and clips are over, it should be taken out immediately
5. For retail meat cuts with bone, label should be fixed near the bone and only one label in a pack for individual customer
6. For pork carcases, label is applied far from the ham and at the front side of the hock
7. For lamb carcases, label is applied on the front side of the shank
8. For beef carcases, label is applied on the vertebral column or rib cage or chine bone and for veal carcases, it is on the leg

Post-mortem (PM) inspection procedure

- Head, viscera (organs) and carcase are examined while these move on rails in synchronized manner
- While moving forward on rail, the head and organs of a specific animal should precede its carcase
- Palpation of organs, incision of muscle if deemed essential, smelling the tissues and conducting laboratory examinations if required
- Carcases should not touch each other while moving down the rails to avoid contamination

PM examination of cattle carcase

1. Head

- Exterior sides and eyes are examined first and then, gums, lips and tongue are looked for any signs of foot & mouth disease (FMD), actinomycosis actinobacillosis, necrosis and stomatitis
- Internal and external masseter muscles are incised parallel to lower jaw to detect for *C. bovis* cysts
- To detect actinobacillosis, tuberculosis and abscesses, retropharyngeal, submaxillary and parotid lymph nodes are cut opened
- As tuberculosis bacteria, *Salmonella* and *Yersinia* are naturally found on the cattle and pigs tonsils, it should be taken out and not to be used for edible purpose

- Tonsils are categorised as specified risk material (SRM) on account of BSE and therefore, should be condemned

Lymph nodes

Lymph nodes are inspected chiefly to detect TB

2. Viscera (Offals)

Lungs

- After normal inspection, palpation is done to rule out many diseases like pleurisy, pneumonia, TB, fascioliasis, hydatid cysts, *etc.*

Heart

- Pericarditis, haemorrhages, etc, can be detected by the pericardium examination
- Particular attention should be given on the endocardium to detect petechial haemorrhages, cysticerci and hydatid cysts
- A flabby condition of the myocardium normally indicates septicaemia in cow

Liver

- Normal observation with palpation should be made for fatty change, actinobacillosis, abscesses, and presence of flukes, hydatidiosis and *C. bovis*
- Liver should not be condemned if infested with liver fluke

Oesophagus, stomach and intestines

- Examine closely and touch the organs with firm hand (palpation)
- The inner (serous) sides may reveal TB or actinobacillosis lesions
- Foreign body may be present in the front part of the reticulum

Kidney

- Kidneys are enucleated for close examination
- Kidneys and associated lymph nodes are incised if required

Spleen

- Visually, it is examined, palpated and cut open if required for any evidence of TB, haematomata and infarcts

Uterus

- Visually, it is examined, palpated and cut open if required
- Signs of past parturition or present pregnancy - non significant
- It should not be incised/touched if the animal is brucella reactor

Udders

- Harbour food-poisoning microorganisms- so questionable for edible purpose
- It should be examined by palpation and every portion of udder and related lymph nodes are incised and observed for septic mastitis and abscesses
- Supramammary lymph nodes should be cut opened for presence of abscesses or TB lesions
- If the animal is brucella positive, it is incised as a whole without opening and carried away without direct touching

Testes (fries)

- Visual examination followed by palpation if intended for edible purpose

3. Carcase

- Visual examination is carried out for carcase surfaces, pleura, peritoneum, diaphragm and incised areas of muscles and bones
- Special observation should be made regarding nutritional status of carcase, bleeding efficiency, odour, colour, carcase hygiene, bruises and any other defects of the carcase
- Palpate and incise the muscles/areas if it is required *e.g. triceps brachii* in case of *C. bovis*
- Visual examination and if necessary, followed by palpation and incision of lymph nodes such as external and internal iliac, renal, superficial inguinal and prepectoral lymph nodes
- If the animal is tuberculin reactors and assumed to be suffering from systemic TB and pathological findings were detected in various organs, its major lymph nodes must be inspected
- Both thoracic and abdominal cavities should be examined for evidence of actinobacillosis, TB, inflammation and abscesses
- If in the animals of that area, occurrence of *Cysticercous cellulosae* is high, tongue base and external masseter muscles must be cut opened and palpated

Post-mortem examination of large animal calves

- Performed similar to adult large animals with particular consideration to special areas
- Mouth and tongue are viewed carefully- for the lesions of FMD and calf diphtheria
- Abomasum and small intestine are visually examined for lesions of peptic ulcer and white scour/dysentery, respectively
- Liver, portal lymph nodes and posterior mediastinal lymph nodes are examined for congenital TB
- Lungs, kidneys and spinal cord are observed to detect melanin deposits and the umbilicus and joints are visually examined for the septic omphalophlebitis--- by noting the colour and viscosity of synovial fluid from hock joint
- Observations are made regarding renal fat colour and consistency

Post-mortem examination of sheep and goats

- These animals need less extensive examination compared to other animals including large animals
- The usual examination does not need any incisions

Post-mortem examination of pigs

- Similar to large animal post-mortem examination
- Skin is carefully observed as classical lesions of swine erysipelas, swine fever and urticarial are visible
- The skin should also be observed for 'shotty eruption', the tail for necrosis, the legs for abscess and the udder for actinomycosis
- Regularly, submaxillary lymph nodes are inspected for TB lesions
- If *Cysticercus cellulosae* is widespread, inspect the muscle from outer side especially the muscles of thigh including heart, tongue, diaphragmatic pillars, the intercostal muscles as well as larynx
- When trichinosis is prevalent, careful inspection and microscopic examination of muscles should be performed
- Submaxillary and supramammary lymph nodes are regularly cut opened for examination in sows
- The mesenteric lymph nodes of pigs are no longer incised because of the frequent contamination of knives with *Salmonella* organisms which may be present in the nodes

- *Salmonella* is commonly found in the mesenteric lymph nodes of pigs and hence, it is not incised because of fear of knives being infected with it

Decisions at post-mortem examination

- The three important decision taken during PM examination are
    1. Permitted for human consumption
    2. Complete condemnation for human consumption
    3. Partly condemned for human consumption—meat for Freibank system or inferior quality meat
- Normally, if the animal is suffering from the *acute* and *generalised* disease, whole carcase and the viscera will be *totally condemned* whereas, in case of *chronic* and *localised* disease condition, *local condemnation* or in few instances *no condemnation* at all
- Total condemnation in cases of actinobacillosis (acute case), actinomycosis (generalized), advanced form of anaemia, anthrax, black leg, *Cysticerous bovis* (generalized), *Cysticerous cellulose*, FMD, metritis, glanders *etc.*
- The ultimate decision regarding a carcase or viscera is taken by considering all the evidences gathered during PM examinations by inspections, palpation, incision, smell and observations made during ante-mortem inspection as well as laboratory results

Declare unfit the entire carcase, viscera and blood of animal showing signs of the disease. This comprises:

i. If the animal has not went through ante-mortem examination excluding wild game slaughtered by hunting
ii. If the animal has not went through post-mortem examination
iii. If the animal dies before slaughter, stillborn animal, foetus and animal slaughtered within 7 days of birth
iv. If the animal is affected with diseases mentioned in OIE List A or B but not in Section IV
v. If the animal is suffering from generalized form of conditions like septicaemia, pyaemia, toxaemia or viraemia
vi. If the slaughtered meat samples does not meet microbiological standards
vii. If the meat sample is infested with parasites which are not mentioned in Section IV

viii. If the meat samples show residues/contaminants level exceeding the maximum permissible level set by the authorities
ix. If the meat samples contain drug residues of illegal compound or treated with illegal compound
x. If the animal age is more than 2 years and belongs to region affected with heavy metals, liver and kidneys of such animal is condemned
xi. If the animal is treated illicitly with disinfecting agents
xii. If the animal is exposed illicitly to irradiation or UV rays
xiii. If foreign bodies are found in animal excluding bodies that are used to hunt the game animal
xiv. If the meat/offal exhibits radioactivity more than the permissible legal levels
xv. If the animal carcase is detected with physiological abnormalities such as change in meat texture, poor bleeding barring in case of game animal or change in flavour such as intense sex odour
xvi. If the animal is emaciated
xvii. Contains specific risk material, except as provided for under Community legislation
xviii. If the animal carcase parts or any offal is classified as specific risk material by Community laws
xix. If the animal carcase parts or any offal is contaminated with soil, faeces or other things
xx. If the animal is suffering from some specific disease or blood gets infected during collection making its blood a public safety concern, its blood is declared unfit
xxi. In the opinion of the official veterinarian, after examination of all the relevant information, it may constitute a risk to public and animal health or is for any other reason not suitable for human consumption
xxii. if the veterinary doctor, after going through all the reports of AM inspection, PM inspection and laboratory report, concludes that animal meat may pose public and animal health threat

The regulation Annex I, Section IV, Chapter IX also recognizes six following particular diseases/infestations for which special guidelines are provided

1. Transmissible Spongiform Encephalopathies (BSE and Scrapie)

- In a region where BSE is prevalent, specific risk materials such as brain, spinal cord or any nervous tissue are condemned
- Also, specific risk materials from normal slaughtered animal is not fed to any animal

2. Cysticercosis

- *Taenia solium – C. cellulosae* – human pork tape worms
- If meat is infested at more than one place with *C. bovis*, it is declared not fit for edible purpose
- If meat is infested at only one area, the carcase parts not infested might be declared fit for edible purpose provided it undergoes cold treatment at lower than -7 °C for minimum 3 weeks or -10 °C for minimum 2 weeks

3. Trichinellosis

- Roundworm *Trichinella spiralis* affects pig, rat, man and many mammals
- Man gets infested by consuming poorly cooked port or its different products like sausages, ham and salami
- Testing meat for *Trichinella* and cold treatment of infested meat may render it safe
- The meat thickness determines the time duration and temperature for cold treatment

4. Glanders

- The serous membrane of the trachea, larynx, nasal cavities and sinuses are closely examined
- If the horse is suffering from glanders, meat is declared unsuitable for edible purpose

5. Tuberculosis

- Consumption of meat of TB affected large ruminants has not ever been recorded to infect human
- Animals that are positive to an intradermal tuberculin test are slaughtered separately and that precautions are taken to avoid cross-contamination
- Tuberculin positive food animals are slaughtered at different area to prevent spread of infection

- If PM examination shows *generalised* TB lesions affecting more than one offals or carcase part, the entire carcase, its organs as well as blood must be classified as not fit for human consumption
- If PM examination reveals *localised* TB lesions affecting only one offal or carcase area, only the infected offal or carcase area is condemned

6. Brucellosis

- In case of acute brucellosis, carcase, offals and blood must be declared unsuitable for edible purpose

Common post-mortem findings

Abscesses

- Most frequently observed pathological findings in pigs
- The main bacterium involved in all abscesses is *Actinomyces pyogenes*

Decision taken if abscesses are found in pig body during PM examination

- *Abscesses at one place*: Normally affected area is declared unfit and rest of the carcase and offals are declared fit after close inspection
- *Abscesses located at tail and on the spinal column*: Affected body part is trimmed *i.e.* tail and the spinal column
- *Abscesses at tail and in the lungs, ribs, peritoneum or forelegs*: Whole carcase is declared unfit for consumption
- *Abscesses in the tail and hind leg*: Removal of the affected parts are enough

Omphalophlebitis or navel ill

- This is a routinely encountered in countries where practice of slaughter of 4–8 days old calves is normally done
- If the condition is systemic (affecting umbilical vessels) whole carcase along with offals is condemned but in case of localised infection affecting only the umbilicus, only affected part is removed

Arthritis

- Finding slightly red coloured synovial fluid in the joints is neither uncommon nor important
- Though, to safe-guard the public and maintain aesthetic appearance, the decisions can be taken based on below given facts:
  - If pus is found in the joint, the limb must be removed to the joint above the one showing the lesions

- The whole limb is discarded in case iliac, prescapular/prepectoral lymph nodes are also affected
- If lymphatic system of 3 or more limbs is infected, the carcase requires condemnation
- If the iliac lymph node is not affected but the popliteal lymph node is swollen, only the lower limb is discarded
- In case of systemic or acute arthritis, the whole carcase as well as offals are declared unfit

Oedema

- It is of less serious concern if it is localised or oedema of insignificant type, ascites and hydrothorax compared to anasarca
- In *anasarca* (oedema) affecting the subcutaneous and connective tissues or oedema leading to emaciation and carcase not showing rigor mortis must be classified as unfit for human consumption

Pneumonia and pleurisy

- If PM inspection reveals systemic involvement of offals, whole condemnation is warranted
- If the condition is localised, trimming of the affected pleura or discarding the rib cage will serve the purpose
- If the pleura is removed, the diaphragm must be discarded in all the cases

Endocarditis

- Whole carcase is considered unfit for human condemnation

Bruising

- Bruised area is trimmed off to satisfy the aesthetic value

Pigmentation

- If pigment origin is from the exterior of the body, it is called exogenous pigments and if it originates from within the body, it is called endogenous pigments
- Exogenous pigments gain entry inside animal body if they graze on land polluted by factories and municipalities
- The frequently encountered pigment is carbon/coal dust which is found as black elements in the lungs and its related lymph nodes
- Xanthophyll and carotenoid pigments originating from carotene A and B are of plant origin

- These lipochrome pigments are frequently found in various body parts of a food animal

Melanin

- Melanin, brownish-black protein, is synthesized by melanocytes using tyrosine amino acid by oxidation and it is found in pigmented skin tissue of an animal
- Mainly bovines and rarely sheep and pig shows unusual melanin deposits called melanosis
- Offals affected with melanin deposits are considered unfit for consumption but melanin is not injurious
- If melanosis affects the whole body, entire carcase is discarded
- Melanomas, a type of malignant tumours, are caused by melanin producing cells called melanocytes
- If melanoma is found during PM examination, a careful inspection of whole carcase is carried out and if the condition is metastasis, total condemnation is recommended

Haematogenous pigments

- In few unusual cases, pigments from haemoglobin breakdown are found in the carcase

Haematin

- It is encountered in conditions where there is extensive breakdown of RBCs such as babesiosis

Haemosiderin

- Pigment haemosiderin joins with ferritin and appears brown or black
- Sometimes, such pigment gets accumulated in the kidneys of Angora goat and give look of enamelled jewellery –*cloisonné kidney*

Icterus

- When formation of bilirubin exceeds its excretion from body due to haemolysis during obstructive liver or toxic reasons, it results in icterus body called jaundice or hyperbilirubinaemia
- It results in distinct yellow colour of surficial fat, fat adhered to offals and serous membranes
- Jaundice must be differentiated from normal yellow colour of fat encountered in case of old cattle and few breeds such as in Jerseys and Guernseys

- This normal yellow colour is due to accumulation of carotene derived from grass
- In such normal cases, yellowness is observed only in fat tissue as carotene pigment is soluble only in fat
- Carcase showing icterus must be examined under natural daylight as the artificial light may alter the true colours
- Complete rejection of whole carcase is required if the icterus is present in carcase even if it is detained for 24 h
- Such type of cases are due to obstructive jaundice where there is extensive haemolysis

Laboratory tests for icterus

Fat (2 g) from the doubtful sample is mixed with 5 ml of a 5% NaOH sol. & boiled for 1 min

↓

Cooling followed by addition of ether (3–5 ml)

↓

Shaking & allowed to stand

↓

Layers will separate

↓

Appearance of greenish-yellow colour in the upper layer---carotenoid pigments

Appearance of greenish-yellow colour in the bottom layer--- bile pigments

Porphyrin

- Porphyrins are a set of red colour elements of iron-bearing haem which forms the haemoglobin pigment
- The porphyrias are a set of syndromes distinguished by extensive porphyrins or their precursors formation in the tissues resulting from alteration in haem synthesis due to enzymatic deficiencies
- Porphyrias is characterized by skin crumbliness and blisters, stomach pain, paralysis, anaemia, teeth and bones turning reddish-brown and even death in acute cases
- The production of photodynamic porphyrins and other substances in the blood results in photosensitisation causing dermatitis and oedema
- Photosensitisation causes formation of porphyrias lesions which are restricted to skin areas which are white, pigment less and low hairy which becomes red and oedematous
- Commonly affected parts are the face and ears, but teats, vulva and perineum may also be involved.

- Face and ears are usually affected areas, however, vulva, teats and peritoneum too show lesions
- If it is affecting a localized area, only that part is rejected

Tumours

- An unusual uncontrolled increase in new cell mass which is not as per the normal growth is called tumour or neoplasm
- If the animal is healthy and the tumour is of benign in nature, only involved part or offal is discarded
- If tumours presence is found in various parts and offals, it requires complete rejection

Poor condition/emaciation

- Leanness and emaciation show body condition differing only in level of degree but the etiology of both might be the same
- Emaciation is caused by some diseases like TB and Johne's disease in large ruminants and gastroenteritis by parasites, chronic fasciola infestation and caseous lymphadenitis in sheep characterized by wasting of muscle
- Similarly, in pigs, swine fever, paratyphoid and erysipelas, can cause muscle wasting due to extended off feeding
- Skin *tenting test* is performed by pulling up a part of the skin with two fingers and allowed to retain the original shape
- In emaciated animal, it takes more the 45 seconds to retain its original shape
- Emaciation is characterized by loss of body fat and its consistency is changed
- Usual fat deposits found in mesentery, mediastinum, omentum, perirenal fat, subcutaneous fat and inter- and intramuscular fat become contracted showing unusual yellowish look having jelly-like consistency
- Proximate analysis of such meat shows lower fat, protein and minerals contents and higher water
- In exceptionally emaciated animals, meat may contain water up to 80% with a protein level of around 19%, thus water to protein ratio reaching at over 4: 1
- An emaciated carcase looks moist externally and in the body cavities and advent of rigor-mortis is abnormal

- Alteration in fat consistency is most prominently observed near the heart base, in the mediastinum, around kidneys or amid the spinous processes of the vertebral column
- Final judgement depends on the extent of body waste, carcase setting efficiency, existence of disease and laboratory tests reports

Based on body health status, decisions that could be taken are given below

1 Fit for edible purpose provided that meat should be supplied to limited areas
2 Little abnormality in meat but suitable for human consumption
3 On economics basis, the carcase after undergoing heat treatment is declared fit for edible purpose
4 Whole carcase must be rejected if the emaciation is due to chronic infection and lab reports have proved it or it has revealed presence of antimicrobials or drug residues

Contamination

- The biggest hazard come across during PM examination is the contamination of carcase with faeces
- This happens due to highly dirty animal or improper bunging or due to rupture of abdomen during dressing
- It is recommended to trim the soiled part affected with such contamination (purulent discharge, bile or faeces)

Parasitic conditions

Ascaris suum

A. suum is roundworm of pigs whose larvae causes classical white spots on the liver while migration making it unsuitable on aesthetic ground

Echinococcus granulosus: Hydatidosis and hydatid cyst

- Dog tapeworm with domestic and wild ruminants acting as intermediate hosts
- Carefully remove the cyst from the organ

*Taenia hydatigena (*in larval stage, it is referred as *Cysticercus tenuicollis)*

- Intestinal dog tapeworms of largest size
- Sheep, cattle, pig and horse act as intermediate hosts of cysticerci
- In these animal, its predilection sites is liver as well as abdominal cavity

- The diameter of fully developed *Cysticercus tenuicollis* is nearly 5–8 cm and it appears on the peritoneum as 'bladder worms'

***Fasciola hepatica:* Liver fluke**

- The immature flukes migrate in the parenchyma of live creating tunnel like shapes and thus damaging it
- During the wet months, this injury can be quite widespread turning the liver visually unfit for consumption

Courses of action

Various factors such as disease prevalence, economic impact, availability of the heat treatment facility for conditionally approved meat, influences the final judgement delivered after PM examination in different countries. The following major conclusions are drawn:

1. Approved for human consumption
2. Totally condemned
3. Partially condemned

Conditionally approved for human consumption

- In few countries, if meat is supposed to be harmful for human/animal or carcase meat is hygienically unacceptable, it is treated under heat or freezing under official observation so as to make it harmless for food

Approved for human consumption, with distribution restricted to limited areas

- If meat is quite costly in a region or it is from animals quarantined due to disease outbreak
- In these conditions, public safety should not be compromised at all and meat must not go beyond the limited area to contain the disease

Freibank meat

- In few countries such as Germany, carcases are classified into three after PM inspection such as:

  I. Meats "passed" for unrestricted sell

  II. Freibank meats- carcases allowed to be sold under certain restrictions, and

  III. Carcases which are condemned and unfit for consumption

- Freibank meats comprises of all meats which could barely be permitted for sell without restrictions and in fresh condition

- They are allowed to be sold due to high economic value of the meat and sold only to people who could not afford the premium quality meat
- It is also to utilize the high value meat protein which would otherwise be wasted if not allowed under Friebank system
- Only a restricted quantity is sold to a household
- Friebank meat must be sold after suitable treatment of suspected meat to make it safe for the public

Hazard analysis and critical control points (HACCP) System

- For effective implementation of an HACCP system both the in-house quality assurance staff and the regulatory authority must work in coordinated manner
- Critical control points (CCPs) should be of limited number in an HACCP system to make it simpler and monitoring less complex and there must be adequate suppleness so as to bring the required changes

HACCP system involves the successive steps given below

1. Hazard Analysis
2. Determination of the CCPs
3. Establish critical limits
4. Establish a system to monitor control of the CCP
5. Corrective action
6. Verification
7. Documentation

1. Hazard analysis

- The initial step to implement the HACCP in a meat processing plant is to recognise and enumerate the different hazards and risks (suck as microbiological, physical and chemical) during the processing steps

The following terminologies are significant

i. **Hazard:** any biological, chemical or physical cause in/state of meat having with the possibility to be harmful to human health

ii. **Severity:** the seriousness (magnitude) of the hazard

iii. **Risk:** an estimate of the likely occurrence of a hazard

- To find out the hazard, severity and risk within a meat processing line, different expert persons like meat microbiologists, line engineers, veterinarians, sanitation experts *etc.* are required

- The various steps of processing are deeply examined and minimum regulatory standards starting from the raw materials to the final products are scrutinized

2. Determination of the CCPs

- CCP is a point in any process (either product preparation/cleaning) at which control can be applied and it is essential to avoid or destroy the hazard or to bring it down to a satisfactory level
- Selection of an effective and necessary CCP is very important for a impactful HACCP program otherwise it may lead to selection of too many insignificant CCPs
- To select an effective and genuine CCP, a decision tree is prepared

3. Establish critical limits

- Critical limit is a standard to differentiate acceptable from unacceptable
- Critical limit should be quantitative in nature instead of qualitative which helps in recognizing if the processing is under control or not
- Quantitative criteria can be measured and specify conclusively whether the system is running under control or not
- Examples of quantitative criteria: time, temperature, pH and chemicals concentration *etc.*
- Qualitative critera are much harder to measure accurately and so, it is tough to determine the deviation from the set standard. Such criteria are colour, smell *etc.*
- Criteria for microorganism are specifically hard to set in term of quantity

4. Establish a system to monitor control of the CCP

- Monitoring is checking a particular CCP to determine whether the CCP is under control or not
- Done by the workers involved or by supervisors
- This is best carried out by the operatives themselves or by their supervisors rather than by a dedicated quality assurance officials
- This checking should be part of normal routine of the processing line for better quality guarantee and an effective HACCP

5. Corrective action

- Corrective procedures should be indicated if the monitoring of a specific CCP reveals deviations

6. Verification

- Measures should be laid down for verification to ensure efficient implementation of HACCP system
- Verifications are performed sequentially by the quality assurance officials and the veterinary examination team

7. Documentation

- Documentation related to all procedures carried out is must and records all the principles and their application

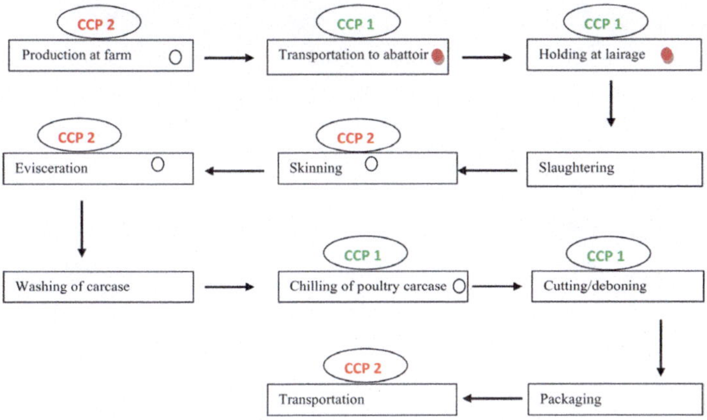

Fig. 6.2. Flow diagram to show CCPs for poultry processing plant. (O) shows a point of minor contamination. (●) shows a point of major contamination; CCP1 indicates effective CCP; CCP2 indicates not absolute CCP (International Commission on Microbiological Safety of Foods (ICMSF)).

7

Slaughtering of Food Animal

Introduction

- **Slaughtering of meat animals in way so as to effect minimum pain and suffering to animals is referred as humane slaughter**
- Slaughtering method followed should inflict least stress and suffering to the animals
- There are acceptable and the unacceptable slaughtering methods and there is no 'nice' method to slaughter the food animals
- In advanced countries, common slaughtering method consists of two steps, stunning and bleeding
- Stunning is done to make animal unconscious and not to feel the pain during actual bleeding process which is followed next
- Exception of stunning-- Jewish and Muslim methods of slaughter

Types of slaughter

Humane slaughter

↓ types of slaughter

- Scientific slaughter
  - ↓ Stunning+ sticking
- Religious (ritual) slaughter
  - ↓ i. Jewish slaughter of slaughter
  - ii. Halal/Muslim method of slaughter
  - iii. *Jhatka* (Sikh) method of slaughter
- Other methods of slaughter
  - ↓ Neck-stab or evernazione method

Stunning

Humane slaughter consists of stunning followed by sticking (bleeding). Stunning is the process of making the animal unconscious till it is slaughtered so that the pain suffered during actual act of slaughtering can be alleviated

Objectives of stunning

i. To bring instant unconsciousness—alleviates pain during bleeding--animal welfare

ii. To make the animal adequately immobile to enable the sticking/bleeding without any struggle—safety to the worker

- It is essential that in the two-step slaughtering process (stunning and then sticking), the unconsciousness is maintained till anoxia is achieved by bleeding making the loss of sensibility irrevocable
- Maintaining unconsciousness till bleeding is ensured by shortening the time delay between stunning and sticking, and it also depends on the efficiency of the exsanguination process
- Satisfactory bleeding can occur where cardiac arrest has been induced if the act of bleeding process is initiated within 3 min of cardiac arrest
- This provides the possibility of outright killing the animal by stunning instead of only making it unconscious
- This removes the unintentional cruelty mated out to animal during slaughtering
- Besides ensuring the welfare of animals, stunning also ensures safety to workers involved in sticking (bleeding) and subsequent shackling as it renders animals immobile

Permitted methods of stunning for ruminants, pigs and solipeds

1. Mechanical methods- e.g. captive bolt
2. Electrical stunning
3. Gas stunning
    - Use of puntilla, hammer or poleaxe is prohibited

Confirming insensibility of animals at the time of slaughter

- Using nervous system consisting of
    - Brain and spinal cord (central nervous system)
    - The peripheral nerves-- vital regulator and communication system
- The brain, comprising of cerebellum and medulla oblongata, the two cerebral hemispheres, is accountable for harmonizing the different important activities of life

Stunning-- a state of unconsciousness or insensibility produced to ensure that the animal does not feel pain during bleeding (sticking) which is generally followed by instant exsanguination

The time gap between exsanguination and insensibility is influence by

- Bleeding technique used
- The species of animal
- Animal age
- Position of the carcase (suspended or horizontal)

Time taken to achieve 'brain death' in

- Sheep - 2–7 sec
- Pigs - 12–30 sec (usually 18 sec)
- Cattle -20–102 sec (average 55 sec).
- Variations are because of changes in the arteries supplying blood to brain through the Circle of Willis

Typical signs of effective stunning

i. Typical signs of effective stunning by electricity --- called ***Electroplectic fits***
ii. Typical signs of an effective stunning using concussive methods
iii. Typical signs of effective stunning using carbon dioxide gas

***i. Typical signs of effective stunning by electricity* --- Electroplectic fits**

- Instant falling of animal with flexion
- Then it leads to stiff extension of the limbs
- Opisthotonus (severe arching back of the neck and spine)
- The eyeballs will roll toward down with tonic (continuous) muscular spasm shifting into clonic (repeated) violent spasms and
- Ultimately, muscle relaxes
  - All the above mentioned signs of effective stunning are together defined as *electroplectic fit*
  - The duration of tonic spasms is about 10–25 sec whereas the clonic phase lasts for 15–45 sec, in sheep as well as pigs
  - Tonic musculor spasm is of shorter duration than clonic spasm
  - Tonic musculor spasm is followed by clonic spasm

ii. The typical signs of an effective concussive stunning

- Instant falling of animal on ground, then tonic spasm for nearly 10–15 sec followed by slow clonic spasm of the hind legs and finally, forceful hind leg movements

- The duration of tonic spasm in pig is short (nearly 3–5 sec) which is instantly succeeded by forceful clonic muscle spasms turning it tough and unsafe for workers to bleed the animal
- Typical rhythmic respiration must stop instantly
- The eyeball should have static gaze with outward look and not face inward

iii. Typical signs of effective stunning using carbon dioxide gas- generally used in pigs or poultry

- The signs of effective carbon dioxide stunning in pigs are those signs similar to observed in chemical anaesthetic and ultimately resulting in loss of consciousness
- Initially, there will be high respiratory rate succeeded by slow respiratory rate and eventually, dyspnoea (difficult breathing) sets in
- Lack of corneal and palpebral reflexes and severe relaxation of muscle
- Ultimately, limbs and jaw become flaccid

Judging the effectiveness of stunning

- Presence or absence of palpebral, corneal and pupillary reflexes do not truly shows the efficiency of the stunning technique
- Animals and birds stunned and then rendered unconscious effectively might display palpebral and corneal reflexes
- Contrarily, an animal might not show palpebral reflex even if it has not been stunned effectively
- Full pupillary dilatation is a dependable sign indicating complete unconsciousness following stunning of an animal
- But this sign is of small utility as the unconsciousness in sheep is ensured 8 sec after the beheading of head and complete pupillary dilatation takes place only 87 sec later
- *The most trusted sign of complete insensibility is the loss of respiratory movement*
- After stunning, reappearance of normal respiratory activity shows regaining of consciousness and must be acted upon
- Presence of irregular breathing gasp is not similar to reappearance of normal respiratory activity and is not of any concern
- Impending brain death is indicated by ‘gagging’ respiratory activities known as agonal breathing

- Normally, vocalisation by animals after stunning during the onset of insensibility is suggestive of pain and distress
- However, lack of vocalisation does not assure absence of pain and distress

Stunning methods

The factors affecting the selection of a specific method of stunning:

- Breed, species, breed and animal age
- Anticipated line speed
- Humane aspects
- Capital and maintenance costs
- Effectiveness of equipment
- Simplicity of operation
- Safety of workers
- Influence on carcase and brain
- Religious and legal necessities

Methods of stunning

Following types of stunning are used for meat animals:

1. Percussive stunning (Captive bolt stunning)
   1.1 Penetrative captive bolt stunning
   1.2 Non-penetrative captive bolt stunning
2. Gas stunning (Exposure to gas mixtures) – CO_2 stunning
3. Electrical stunning

1. Percussive stunning (Captive bolt stunning)

- Known as captive bolt because cartridge never comes out of barrel (remains captive inside the pistol) (Fig. 7.1)
- The bolt is forced frontward by the cartridge and then, it retreats back into the barrel
- Captive bolt pistol is the commonest type of percussive stunner in which bolt is driven outside by blank cartridge and then it returns back mechanically inside the barrel
- Cartridge of correct strength should be applied for the different species

Cartridge strength

- 1 grain for small animals such as milk lambs
- Up to 3 grains for large ruminants and 4 grains for adult bulls (1 grain = 0.065 g)

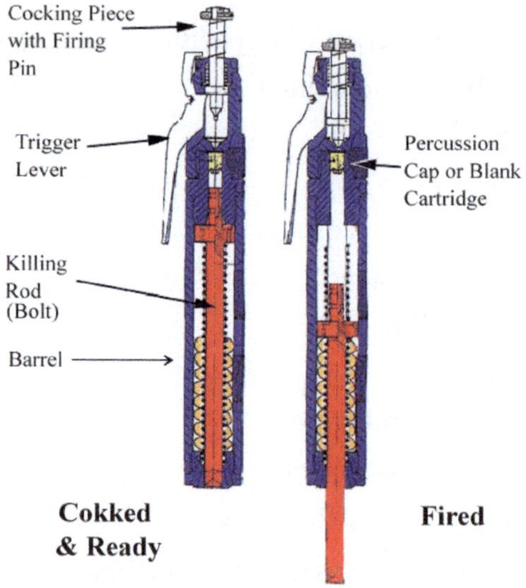

Fig. 7.1. Penetrating captive bolt (Firearms History, Technology & Development, 2011). Firearms History, Technology & Development. (2011). Utility Firearms: Meat Processing Industry, March 11, 2011. Retrieved on 09/09/2024 http://www.firearmshistory.blogspot.com/2011/03/utility-firearms-meat-processing.html)

- Captive bolt stunning is quite effective if applied correctly in matured large ruminants, sheep and calves except in bulls and pigs particularly in boars and sows due to
  - Much thicker frontal bone and
  - Difficulty in restraining and thus pointing the stunner at precise point

1.1 Penetrative captive bolt stunning

- In this type of stunning, the bolt pierces the animal skull bone causing destruction of the brain and then recoils back into the barrel (Fig. 7.2)
- The animal gets stunned during this process due to what is known as acceleration concussion
- Brain is destroyed so cannot be used for human consumption

Acceleration concussion

- Penetrative captive bolt causes instant unconsciousness by
  - The damage of cortex and much inner portion of the brain
  - Changes in intracranial pressure
  - The abrupt jerk to the brain
- **All these brain changes are collectively known as *acceleration concussion***
- In captive bolt pistol, the chief force in bringing insensibility to animals is the impact energy of the bolt which is determined by the bolt speed at which it strikes the brain and not on the depth of destruction of brain

Bolt velocity required

- 55 m/s for large ruminants, steers and heifers
- 65 to 70 m/s for young bulls

Working principle of percussive stunner (captive bolt)

- Percussive stunning brings the desired unconsciousness by imparting impact energy to brain which causes turbulent circular and other movements of the cerebral hemispheres and thus enhances the incidence of collision between the cortex and the skull bone resulting in brain tissue damage
- Above phenomenon brings about diffuse depolarisation and synchronised discharge of cortical neurons.
- Further, direct destruction and shock are produced to the cerebral hemispheres and brainstem by the penetrative percussive stunners
- Due to complicated reloading, slaughter rates of about 240–250 animals/h can be achieved with penetrative percussive stunner
- Produces blood splashing condition in muscle

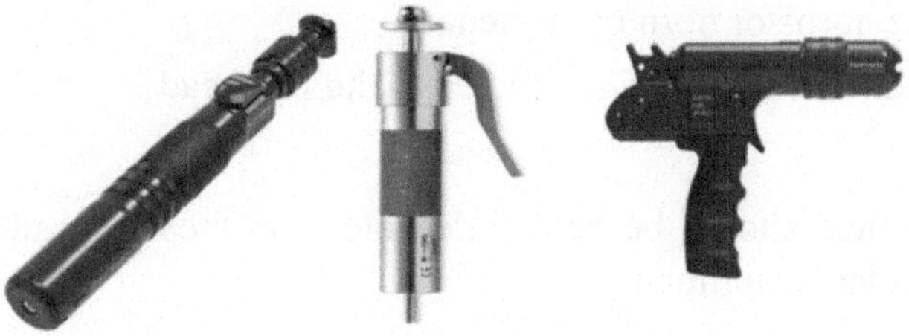

Fig. 7.2. Various types of percussive stunner

Pneumatic stunners

- The bolt is propelled using 80–120 psi pressure
- Complex loading and reloading of cartridge
- Massive bolt velocity is attained under suitable pressure

1.2 Non-penetrative concussion stunners

- Bolt does not pierces through the skull bone
- Bolt having mushroom-fashioned head is utilised in calves and lambs for producing non-penetrative concussion stunning
- This type of stunner is barred by EU Council Regulation to be used on ruminants of more than 10 kg body weight
- Efficient in bringing instant unconsciousness in animals
- Does not produce blood splashing but may produce intracranial haemorrhages in animals having thin frontal bones
- Incidence of blood splashing is not a problem with this type of stunning, however, intracranial bleeding occurs in animals possessing thin frontal bones of skull
- This stunning is used to salvage brain for edible purpose
- Insensibility lasts for 30 s in calves
- In older animal, non-penetrative captive bolt stunning is not used– do not produce enough insensibility

Head sites for percussive stunning (captive bolt stunning)

- The stunner is placed at the right point and direction on the head with firm hands

Cattle

- The proper site in matured cattle is at the centre of forehead at the point of intersection of two lines drawn from the inner canthus of eyes to the opposite horns or horn prominence
- The stunner is held at right angles to the forehead

Calves

- The stunned should be held little below on the forehead compared to matured large ruminants

Bulls & old large ruminants

- They should not be shot at the point of poll

- The stunner muzzle is held 1.5 cm adjacent to the ridge which runs down across the middle of forehead

Sheep & goats

- Stunner is kept on the top of the head pointing towards the gullet in hornless sheep and goat

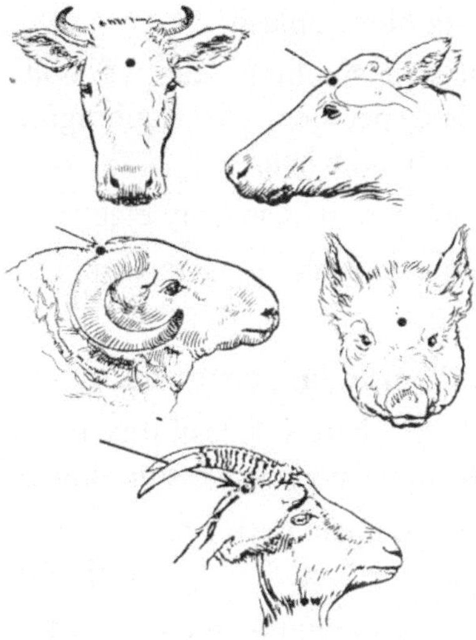

Fig. 7.3. Different head sites for placing concussive stunner in case of matured large ruminants, calves, horned sheep, pigs, horned goats (by courtesy of the Universities Federation for Animal Welfare).

Pigs

- The muzzle is held 2.5 cm above the middle of the line joining the inner canthus of both the eyes and pointed towards the cranial cavity in case of pigs of bacon weight

Older pigs

- In older pigs, frontal bones of skull are big and skull is huge rendering captive bolt stunning less effective
- Hence, the stunner is held firmly adjacent to the ridge at the point 5 cm above the middle of the line joining the inner canthus of both the eyes
- The contact-firing types (a little tap on the site of application) of captive bolt stunner are highly suitable than the stunner with trigger

Disadvantages of captive bolt stunning (percussive stunning)

I. Blood splashing

II. Neural embolism

I. Blood splashing

- Results due to delay in bleeding (sticking) after electrical or penetrative percussive (captive bolt) stunning
- The passing of electric current through the brain causes sudden increase in blood pressure and heart beat as a result of vasoconstriction and so, need arises to instantly perform the sticking to release the blood pressure and thus, preventing blood splash
- Penetrative percussive stunning (captive bolt) -- blood splashing is observed in muscles, specifically in diaphragm, the intercostal muscles, the abdominal wall and the heart
- Incidence more common in head-only electrical stunning
- Occurrence of blood splashing is rare in head-to-back/leg electrical stunning

II. Neural tissue embolism in large ruminants

- With concern to BSE, there is possibility that the emboli produced by brain tissue as a result of percussive stunning could enter edible tissues
- Pneumatically operated penetrative captive bolt stunning results in 2.5–5% of large ruminants affected with neural tissue embolism
- Diaphragmatic lobe of the lung---most frequent site
- Pneumatic stunners---causes fragmentation of brain tissue leading to emboli formation
- Penetrative captive bolt stunning produces emboli from tissues of central nervous system in high numbers in large ruminants and sheep which moves through jugular blood
- In non-penetrating captive bolt stunning, CNS tissue was found in jugular blood in only 2% of animals
- Pithing is known to enhance the chance of neural emboli

Free bullet pistol

- The free bullet pistol is commonly employed to kill horses humanely
- Point of application in horses– site of intersection of two lines from the medial canthus of eyes to the roots of opposite ears
- The site of placing the stunner is same as in case of site of captive bolt pistol
- The stunner is directed little downward the right angle level to the forehead

Water jet stunning

- In this way of stunning, a very thin jet of water is forced on the skull which penetrates it and disintegrate the brain tissue by laceration, crushing and sending shockwaves resulting in instant unconsciousness of animal
- The water jet is created under pressure of 3500–4000 bar and applied at the same site as that of captive bolt piercing the skull within 0.2–0.4 s
- Damage to brain causes seizures
- Meat is said to be of better quality than electrical and CO_2 stunning

2. Gas stunning using carbon dioxide and other gas mixtures

- Mainly used for pig stunning and sometimes poultry
- Carbon dioxide is used at 80% or greater level
- For pig stunning/killing, The European Food Safety Authority suggested the below given gas mixtures:
  - A combination of 30% CO_2 and 60% argon or nitrogen in atmosphere, or
  - 90% argon or nitrogen (or other inert gas) in atmosphere
- In these two cases, the residual oxygen level must not exceed by 2% of its volume
- Exposure period-- minimum of 3 min
- 65-70% CO_2 concentration is most ideal
- Bleeding must be within 30 s
- Pigs regain recovery after 1.5 min of stunning
- The regimes provide insensibility for lower than 50 s and hence, exsanguination should start in 25 s
- Presently, only carbon dioxide is commonly utilised at industrial level for stunning of animals
- 80–95% CO_2 level in atmosphere is used for adequate time period to induce stunning/kill pigs followed by exsanguination
- Use of gas stunning system allows for achieving high line speed in pig slaughterhouse.
- Several pigs can be stunned simultaneously using gas stunning.
- Line speeds of 800 pigs/h can be achieved by gas stunning
- If the concentration is very less
  - Stunning of pigs will be imperfect

- if it is too high
  - Pigs may become rigid and display reflex muscle actions and bleed insufficiently
- If the pigs are exposed for long time
  - Occurrence of skin congestion which turns bluish after scalding

Role of CO_2 in producing stunning

- Respiratory and metabolic acidosis occurs as result of breathing of carbon dioxide
- Acidosis brings down the pH of cerebrospinal fluid (CSF) and neuron and this prevents the neurons activity bringing anaesthesia like effects

The different equipment types used to apply gas mixture

- The various equipment types employed for CO_2 stunnig depends on the required slaughter rate
- The equipment types used for CO_2 stunnig are:
  1. The oval tunnel
  2. Dip lift
  3. Compact CO_2 stunner
  4. Combi-Compact stunner

1. The *oval tunnel*

- Not used now
- Slaughter rate: up to 600 pigs/h
- Pigs are carried on slot conveyor belt through an oval gas tunnel
- Tunnel has slope of 30°downside guiding pigs to the anaesthetising chamber
- At the other end of the tunnel, stunned pigs are shackled, lifted to an overhead rail and stuck for bleeding
- The slot conveyor which carries the pigs has 10 compartments to hold 10 pigs
- This system is used for stunning pigs up to 113 kg weight

2. Dip lift

- Appropriate for pig of any weight and also for calves and sheep
- Involves a cage of size 200 cm long, 70 cm high and 50 cm wide
- The animals are loaded in the cage and lowered to CO_2 pit where it remains in CO_2 air for a fixed duration

- Then the cage comes up mechanically with unconscious animals which are subsequently shackled and bled
- Advantage of the system--several pigs to be stunned simultaneously
- System suitable for low throughput

3. Compact CO_2 stunner

- It involves a horizontally circling device consisting of 4-8 compartments each accommodating one animal
- It revolves in such a way that when one compartment is at the topmost for animal loading, the others are dipped inside the gas chamber for stunning
- After the animal is put in the compartment, it moves down and suspend the pig in gas chamber
- The pigs experience the incremental CO_2 concentration such as first exposure to 10% CO_2 , then 30% for 10 s, 60% for 10 s at third position and more than 90% CO_2 for 20 s at the 4th and 5th position and thereafter, pigs are ejected out of unit
- Ability to stun nearly 600 pigs/h

4. Combi-Compact stunner

- Comparable to 'Compact stunner'
- It allows loading of 3-4 pigs/compartment at a time- group loading
- Pigs suffer lower stress
- If panel equipped with sensor is fitted, the apparatus can be tunred party automated
- The gas chambers must be equipped with device to monitor the CO_2 concentration at each position and issue visible and audio warning if the gas level falls below the mandatory level

Advantages of CO_2 stunning/killing

i. Little noise, need of less worker, carcases are relaxed allowing easy dehairing and dressing

ii. Blood yield is improved by 0.75% since CO_2 raises respiration rate resulting in high blood flow and thus higher bleeding

iii. Muscular haemorrhages are prevented

iv. Incidence of bone fractures decreases to nil

v. Pale soft exudative (PSE) condition-- reduced

3. Electrical stunning

- A pair of tongs is used to pass alternating current (AC) through the animal brain and the heart
- The current causes huge depolarisation of neurons in the brain causing tonic and clonic muscle contractions
- This epilepsy type of activity is similar to unconsciousness and seems to be linked to insensibility
- The epileptic type of activity is stimulated by the discharge of glutamate and aspartate neurotransmitters into the extracellular space in the brain
- This is a revocable process in which animal starts retaining its senses after 40 s of stunning
- Most widely used on pigs but also suitable for sheep and calves

The factors affecting an effective electrical stun are

1. The strength of the electric current--- must be sufficient to make the animal unconscious or kill it by cardiac arrest
2. Current should be used for sufficient duration to affect *electroplectic shock*

   Duration of application of electric stunner:

   7 s for low-voltage apparatus and less than 3 s for high-voltage apparatus
3. The electrodes should be properly placed so that the current will travel via the thalamus and cortex, the chief sensory centres in the forebrain

- The electrical resistance faced by the current due to hair and skin can be reduced by dipping the electrodes in brine solution and maintaining the animal head clean and dry
- The wool on the sheep head enhances the electrical resistance considerably
- Pig head should not be moistened as it will cause the current to pass through the pig skin and not through its brain
- It is important that a required level of current must pass through the brain in quick time to render the animal unconscious
- If too high a voltage---incidences of muscle haemorrhages and broken bones
- If voltage is too low -- the animal may be paralysed but remains conscious
- Electrical current passing via the brain causes vasoconstriction resulting in sudden increase in blood pressure and heart rate and thus, necessitating to bleed the animal without delay to prevent blood splashing

Blood splashing

- Results due to delay in bleeding (sticking) after electrical or penetrative percussive (captive bolt) stunning
- Electrical current passing via the brain causes vasoconstriction resulting in sudden increase in blood pressure and heart rate and thus, necessitating to bleed the animal without delay to prevent blood splashing
- Mostly occurs in penetrative percussive stunning
- Head-to-back/leg electrical stunning does not produce blood splashing
- Penetrative percussive stunning (captive bolt) --- blood splashing is seen in muscles, especially in diaphragm, the intercostal muscles, the abdominal wall and the heart
- Incidence more common in head-only electrical stunning
- Bone fracture is more common with high voltage electrical stunning
- Pig is predisposed for such bone fractures which particularly affects pelvis, scapula, the neck of the femur and the 5th or 6th thoracic vertebrae

Types of electrical stunning

1. Low voltage stunning
2. High voltage stunning
   - 2.1 Head-to-brisket stunning of cattle
   - 2.2 Head to back/leg stunning of pigs and sheep

1. Low-voltage electrical stunning

- Using less than 150 V (75 V) for not less than 7s
- Not recommended now
- For head-only electrical stunning, a least electric current of 250 mA for sheep and lambs and 400 mA for pigs -- to create an effective stunning and placing the tongs at the correct position
- However, practically tongs are not placed ideally so higher recommendations—
  - Sheep- 1.0 A
  - Lambs- 0.6 A
  - Pig- 1.3 A and
  - Large ruminants- 1.5 A

2. High-voltage electrical stunning

- Applying 300 V or more is highly effective compared to low-voltage stunning
- The duration of application -- minimum 3 s
- Pigs stunned on the floor may suffer from fractures of vertebrae and scapula

Head-to-brisket stunning of large ruminants

- High-voltage is used in head-to-brisket stunning
- Electrodes are placed after animals are restrained by neck yoke in specifically constructed stunning pen
- Then, a chin lift raises the chin to which nose contact plate is applied
- AC current of not more than 3.5 A (at 550 V, 50 Hz) is applied for 3 s between the nose and neck yoke
- To cause cardiac arrest, one more electrode is applied between the neck and brisket amid the forelegs of animal
- Unconsciousness and cardiac fibrillation is related to:
    - Gasping and/or rhythmic respiratory activity
    - Revolution of the eyeball in few animals, and
    - Regaining corneal and palpebral reflexes in a few
- These reflexes do not specify regaining of the consciousness and can be overlooked
- These reflexes vanish with time and brain death ensures without the return of consciousness

Head to back/leg stunning of pigs and sheep

- High-voltage electrical stunning can be used for
    - Head-only application as well as
    - Head and back/leg
- In this stunning method, the brain is insensible and cardiac arrest takes place and in turn, brain becomes devoid of blood supply
- The animal is out rightly killed and thus delay between stunning and sticking become insignificant
- If sticking is done within 3 min, the bleeding will be adequate in pigs
- 'Pelt burn' in sheep is associated with this system of stunning
- Does not normally produce blood splashing

- Current of
    - 1.3 A and of 250 V-- for pigs and
    - 1.0 A at 375 V for sheep

Conditions necessary for producing effective stunning using electricity

i. Strength of the electrical current should be sufficient to produce insensibility– so at least current of 250 mA and 75 V should be used
ii. Duration of application of current– should be sufficient to produce effective stunning– at least 10 s
iii. Proper placement of electrodes– this ensures that the current passes via the thalamus and cortex
iv. Immediate bleeding following the stunning to avoid regaining consciousness, muscular haemorrhages

Prevention of muscular haemorrhages due to electrical stunning

- Adequate rest to animals
- Proper positioning of electrodes
- Quick bleeding after the stunning
- Efficacy of electrical stunning depends on total quantity of electrical strength applied and does not depends on voltage, duration of application or amperage

Effects of stunning on meat quality

1. Blood splashing
2. Bone fracture

- Gas stunning using CO_2 results in least cases of PSE and blood splash and it largely improves the meat quality
- Similarly, head-to-back/leg electrical stunning causes very few cases of blood splashing
- High voltage electrical stunning- chances of fracture of bones – because of violent tonic fits stimulated during and instantly after stunning
- Bone fractures are commonly observed in pigs in the scapula, pelvis, the neck of the femur and near the 5th or 6th thoracic vertebrae

Other methods of slaughter

1. Neck-stab or evernazione method

- Neck-stab or evernazione method of slaughter is practised in large animals in Mexico, Spain, parts of Italy and some South American countries
- A small double-edged knife (puntilla) is inserted into the occipitoatlantal space at the nape of the neck thus, splitting the medulla oblongata
- It does not produce insensibility and only makes the animal effectively immobile
- The method is condemned-- animals show a photomotor reflex --- suggestive of brain sensibility

2. In the Arctic, curved single edged knife is plunged into occipitoatlantal space of reindeer and pushed further ahead to disintegrate the brain

3. The Sikh/Jakta method

- Decapitation of sheep or goat is performed with one stroke of a sword

Slaughter of poultry

1. Electrical stunning
   1.1 Handheld head-only stunning
   1.2 Electric water baths
2. Gas stunning
3. Percussive stunning of poultry
4. Other methods of slaughter of poultry
   4.1 Cervical dislocation
   4.2 Decapitation

1. Electrical stunning of poultry

Handheld head-only stunning

- Handheld head-only stunning apparatus should be properly designed to make it fit for intended species and type of the bird
- Stunning devises for birds vary in electrode size, surface area of the bird head making contact with electrode, electrodes impedance and the pressure with which electrodes are applied on bird head
- A current of 240 and 400 mA—for 7 s for poultry and turkeys, respectively, with constant voltage of 110 V & frequency of 50 Hz

- Neck cutting --incising both carotids, within 15 s after the removal of the stunner
- Manually operated stunning devices are only suitable for low rates of kill –
- Hand operated stunners can achieve less slaughter rate (up to 300 chicken/h)

Signs of effective stunning in poultry by handheld head-only stunning

- Firstly, on stunning, there is wing flapping and leg flexion which changes to tonic convulsion, stiff extended legs, rigid arching back of the neck, wings folded firmly round the breast and continued body movement
- Important–properly stunned birds can display reflexes of nictitating membrane and others related to eyes

Electric water baths

- Electric water baths can be utilised to produce stunning as well as killing in birds
- In this method, birds are hanged upside down on proper size shackles and carried over the overhead rail
- While being carried, their heads pass over the electrified water bath touching the water and thus stunning is accomplished
- The shackling is very stressful to the birds
- Wing flapping leads to dislocations and fractures

Assessment of unconsciousness in electrical water bath stunned poultry

- The greatest dependable signs of correctly stunned bird in low-voltage stunning is known as **Electroplectic Fit**
- The features of these signs are the opisthotonus, opened eyes, loss of corneal reflex, wings arched, stiff extended legs and continuous quick body movement
- Inducing cardiac arrest is in favour of animal welfare
- High strength current is reported to cause red skin conditions comprising red wing tips and pyrostyles, haemorrhage of wings, difficult plucking, broken bones (especially the furculum) and ruptured blood vessels resulting in blood splashing of the breast muscle

2. Gas Stunning--Stunning/killing poultry with controlled atmospheres

- Chickens are exposed to gas mixture while being in the transport crates and stunned. Shackling is done later after unconsciousness sets in. This also ensures poultry welfare

The gas mixtures used for poultry

1. Initially, birds are exposed to 40% CO_2, 30% O_2 and 30% N_2 for 1 min during induction phase and subsequently exposed to 80% CO_2 during finishing phase or
2. Birds are kept in air for at least 2 min containing any ratio of argon, nitrogen or any other inert gases with air and CO_2, on the condition that the CO_2 level must not be more than 30% by volume and the residual O_2 is not more than 2% by volume or
3. Birds are exposed for at least of 2 min to gas mixtures containing argon, N_2, other inert gases or any mixture of these gases in air provided that residual O_2 should not be more than 2% by volume

Recommended that

i. At least 2 min exposure should be given to birds to these gas mixtures

ii. After stunning, shackling and bleeding must be completed within 3 min to avoid red wing tips, wing vein engorgement/haemorrhage, shoulder haemorrhage and red feather tracts in broiler carcases

- However, gas stunning produces lower incidence of bone fractures compared to electrical stunning

Advantages of using agron for stunning of poultry

- Exposure to argon causes anoxia and increased drop in muscle pH during the initial hours of post-mortem but does not create condition similar to PSE meat
- If argon is used along with chilling air at 1 °C, filleting can be initiated just after 2 h of slaughter and the sensory attributes of such meat is superior than the control fillets

3. Percussive stunning of poultry birds

- Percussion stunning either penetrative or non-penetrative captive bolt leads to major fractures and injury to skull and brain of the bird

4. Other methods of slaughter of poultry

Cervical dislocation

Usually used at chicken farm and industrial slaughterhouses as standby method

- EU legislation does not permit it
- Does not result in instant unconsciousness but death is due to asphyxiation or ischemia
- Injury to brain tissue results in pain to bird

Likewise,* decapitation *does not produce instant brain insensibility

Effects of stunning on poultry meat quality

- If 50Hz AC is used in water bath stunning and voltage is more than 105 mA for chicken and 150 mA for turkey, it results in fractured bones, internal bleeding in breast and leg muscles deteriorating the carcase quality

Pithing

- Subsequent to stunning of large ruminants using penetrative captive bolt and prior to neck cutting, a long thin rod or coiled wire is inserted into the hole made by the bolt of the stunner
- This action damages the motor centres of the brain causing in loss of muscular reflexes at the time of sticking resulting in safety to worker and increasing the slaughter line speed
- No change in the bleeding level of the carcase
- If the pithing road/wire is longer than 0.6 m, the spinal cord roots of the greater splanchnic nerve which is the main vasoconstrictor of the abdominal cavity, are damaged
- This causes dilatation of the splanchnic blood vessels leading to congestion of the liver, kidneys and intestines as well as congestion and enlargement of the spleen, and this condition is known as '**slaughter spleen'**
- Pithing is very unclean and takes time
- Pithing is not recommended in countries having BSE incidences-Pithing --increased risk of neural emboli

Bleeding

- Just after stunning, bleeding/sticking/exsanguination is performed without delay
- The blood makes 8% of total body weight of the animal
- About 40–60% of the total blood volume comes out by bleeding- avg. 50%

Large ruminants

Two major methods of bleeding of large ruminants

1. Bilateral severance of the carotid arteries and jugular veins by cutting across the throat region behind the larynx similar to ritual slaughter
2. First, a cut is made in the jugular furrow at the base of the neck followed by insertion of the knife towards the entry of the chest to cut the brachiocephalic trunk and anterior vena cava

  - Knife should not be pushed much deeper towards the chest
  - If the pleura is pierced by the deeper knife insertion, blood may go into the thoracic cavity and stick to the parietal pleura, especially along the posterior edges of the ribs
  - This contaminated condition is called **back bleeding or over sticking**

- Bleeding on rail is 40% more effective than those animals bled on floor (horizontally)
- Bleeding time-- 6 minutes in cattle
- About 13.6 kg of blood is drained from large ruminants
- About 1–2.5 kg of blood is drained from sheep
- Bleeding time allowed for sheep is 5 min and
- Blood yield in case of pork pigs, bacon pig and boar and saw is 2.2, 3 and 3.6 kg, respectively
- Blood yield from calves is about 2.7 kg

Bleeding in Sheep/goat

- Bilateral severance is the easiest method to carry out adequate bleeding
- Bilateral severance: Same like large ruminants-- carotid arteries and jugular veins are severed across the throat region behind the larynx similar to ritual slaughter
- Bleeding in horizontal position yields 10% more blood than in vertical position (on rail bleeding)
- Bleeding time in sheep/goat– 5 min

Bleeding (sticking) in pigs

- Sticking is performed in pigs by pushing the knife in the depression found at the anterior of sternum and directed towards the heart to cut the anterior vena cava brachiocephalic trunk at the entry of the chest cavity (at times carotid artery is also cut)
- Knife should not be inserted too deep otherwise it would pierce the shoulder, letting the scalding water and blood to collect beneath the scapula and making this area appear as cooked which is known as **shoulder 'pocket'**
- Bleeding time- 6 min

Prone sticking

- After stunning, the animal is stuck (bled) while lying prone and being conveyed by a conveyor

- A holding-down belt restrains the pigs after sticking to prevent involuntary struggling of pigs
- A trough running though the full length of the conveyor is used to collect the draining blood
- Used in some abattoirs in USA

Advantages of prone sticking

- Efficient recovery of blood
- No broken bones due to struggling & hence no internal ham bruises

Ritual slaughter

1. Jewish method
2. Muslim/Halal method
3. Jhatka/Sikh method

1. Jewish religious slaughter– called Shechita

- **Kosher** is the meat from animals slaughtered as per Jewish law and lawful for them
- **Terefa** is unlawful meat prohibited to be consumed by Jews (opposite to kosher)
- Shechita is the act of animal slaughter as per Jewish law done by **shochet, or cutter** using a very sharp knife called **chalaf**
- **Chalaf** is free from any notch, dent or fault measuring almost double the width of animal's neck and inspected prior to every slaughter
- Washing and curing of meat--- **mehila**
- Except for spinal cord, the four carotid arteries and jugular veins and all the soft tissue structures are cut
- It is important that the cut at the neck is kept extended/opened so that the edges of the cut do not touch each other. This is said that it would avert any pain to animal
- The **five principles of Jewish ritual slaughter**, are that the neck severence shall be performed
  - Without pause, pressure, stabbing, slanting or tearing
- The animal is slaughtered by **shochet ('cutter')** who is helped by a sealer (**shomer**) accountable for placing the kosher mark on the brisket and on edible offal
- The shochet says prayers before slaughter and performs 'post-mortem examination' by placing a cut posterior to the xiphoid cartilage and

putting his hand to sense any adhesions in the thoracic cavity. This act is called '**searching**'

- **Porging**- Removal of major blood vessels
- Usually, forequarters portion is consumed and hindquarters is avoided as it is said that it possess more than 50 blood vessels which requires highly trained kosher butchers for its removal (porging)
- Prior stunning of animals is forbidden
- The persistence of corneal and palpebral reflexes and also the convulsion which occurs after the neck has been severed is not associated with consciousness of animal

2. Muslim methods of slaughter

- This method is quite similar to Jewish method of slaughter and several slaughter practices and rules related to meat consumption are similar in both faiths
- Animal welfare is taken into account during both slaughter practices
- Animals awaiting slaughter should be given feed and water and slaughtering should not be done in front of other waiting animals
- Consumption of meat of pig and dead animals including blood of any animal is prohibited
- Pronouncing the name of Allah is must and slaughterer must be a Muslim
- Using a sharp knife to severe the skin of neck is considered nearly painless and quick loss of blood is said to bring instant insensibility
- Different from Shechita which is administered and controlled by a central board, Muslim method of slaughter is overseen by the local Islamic authority

3. Jhatka/Sikh method

- Decapitation at one stoke of the knife
- Bleeding is said to be less efficient

8

Utilization of Slaughterhouse Byproducts

Fat

- Utmost significant slaughterhouse byproduct is fat obtained from intestines, kidneys, channel and other offals
- Edible ox fat is rendered and the obtained product is called premier jus (higher grade fat) which is differentiated into oleo oil and oleo stearin
- If all edible ox fat is rendered, it is called dripping and it used for human consumption
- Inedible fat is used for soap manufacturing
- The highest value fat from pig is recovered from peritoneal lining (leaf fat), and the subsequent highest value recovered from back fat, mesentery and omentum
- Sheep fat is separated into oleo oil and oleo stearin because of its strong flavour
- Mutton fat is harder and its stearin content is more than ox or pig and therefore, it is applied on the top of meat paste glass jar as a protective layer

Rendering of edible fat

Three principal procedure of rendering of edible fat are:

i. Wet rendering
ii. Dry rendering
iii. Continuous low-temperature rendering

i. Wet rendering

- In the pressure batch cooker type, chopped raw materials are loaded and steam is injected to attain a temperature of 140 °C and pressure for 3-4 h
- Thereafter, pressure is gradually reduced and the fat is collected
- Fat is filtered and centrifuged to obtain fat, water and fines

ii. Dry rendering

- Steam is used to melt the fat loaded in double jacketed vat at atmospheric pressure
- Steam never comes in direct contact with the raw material
- Pressure is build up due to release of moisture
- Process takes 1.5-2 h
- Fat is collected and then filtered and clarified as discussed above

iii. Continuous low-temperature rendering

- Cooking, separation and cooling of finished product takes place in continuous manner
- Ideal process of rendering
- Steam at 90 °C is used to heat the fat
- Fat is centrifuged to remove the fines from the fat
- Process is continuous-- separation of liquid from solid, centrifugation, pressing and drying of solids are continuous
- Fat should be rendered at temperature at which lipase could not get activated
- Lipase gets activated at temperature between 40-60 °C and above 60 °C, it gets inactivated

Processing of stomach

Preparation of tripe

- Stomach are emptied and washed
- Scalding in soda water, scraping followed by cleaning in cold water
- Finally, cooking at 49-60 °C for 3-3.5 h
- 40-45% of the fresh weight (green weight) of stomach is obtained as tripe after the processing

Processing of inedible blood

- BOD of whole blood is 250000 mg/litre
- So, it should not be mixed with waste water
- Whole blood has two components: plasma (60-70%) and red blood cells (RBC) (20-40%)
- Plasma is composed of water (91%) and protein (7-8%)
- RBC contains 34-38% protein and 62% water
- RBC portion used to prepare black sausage or dried to prepare meal

Inedible blood is converted into blood meal by dry rendering by removing water in three ways:

1. Single stage drying- dried to 8-10% moisture level
2. Batch coagulation of blood; followed by draining of serum, pressing the solid to remove moisture and then solid mass is dried
3. Precooking, coagulation and separation using continuous process and finally drying

Processing of hoof and horns

- Hoofs are detached from feet by immersing it in hot water and thereafter, pulling it out
- Hoofs are used to prepare combs and buttons
- Alternatively, steam drier is used to dry and then ground into hoof meal fertilizer
- Combs, hairpins, button and knife handles are made from horns
- Lower grade horns are also turned into fertilizer by grinding

Neatsfoot oil

- Is used as lubricant for delicate machinery

Extraction process of neatsfoot oil

Large ruminants feet

↓

Washing, scalding at 77 °C to ease removal of hairs from feet

↓

Boiling for 15 min to facilitate claws removal

↓

Splitting the feet into two

↓

Long cooking in water

↓

Settling

↓

Supernatant oil is skimmed off

↓

Filtration

↓

Neatsfoot oil

Hair and bristle

- Large ruminants hair are obtained from tannery where lime is used to remove hair from the hides/skins

- Therefore, it needs to be treated with HCl to remove lime, other materials and then sterilized
- Dried cattle hairs are very soft and used as felt for placing beneath the carpet

Bristles

- Mainly obtained from pig back and tail
- Hardest bristles are obtained from wild pigs
- For making various kinds of brushes such as shaving brush

Hides and skins

- Previously, they were the highest valued byproduct obtained from the animal carcase but in last few years their prices have fallen owing to low demand
- Carcase, hide and other byproducts fetch 80, 12 and 7% of total value of the food animal, respectively
- Ox hide is 10% of the carcase weight or 7% of the live weight of the animal
- Grass-fed cattle hide is heavier than stall-fed cattle hide
- Chrome tanning is used to process the hide to obtain leather
- Sole leather is the leather prepared from the animal's butt area
- Sheep skins are converted into chamois leather by 'shammoying' process in which fish oil is applied on the skin to make it soft and pliable

Treatment of condemned meat & offals

Freibank system (basso macello)

- Selling meat of inferior quality and meat which require some treatment before sale
- Such meat is sold under strict governmental/municipal control
- Means to provide nutritious, safe and cheap meat to lower segment of the population
- Only small quantity is given to one person
- Butchers, hotel and restaurants are not allowed to take such meat

Processing of Freibank meat

- Cysticerci and trichinae parasites will be killed if meat is treated at 77 °C
- Boiling of meat pieces not more than 10 cm in diameter for 2.5 h will destroy parasites and effectively inactivate most forms of non-sporing bacteria including tubercle bacilli

- Steam sterilization of meat of up to 15 cm diameter—under pressure of 0.49 kgf/cm^2 for 2 h
- Meat from anthrax, malignant oedema, tetanus, salmonella or septic condition—no treatment is satisfactory—meat must be condemned

Processing of inedible animal byproducts

- The preparation of bone meal and meat-and-bone meal from such materials and feeding these to animals are not recommended as salmonella and anthrax have been reported to spread from feeding such contaminated feeds
- Additionally, handling of such contaminated feed at the rendering plant also poses problem for the workers
- To control the illegal trade of condemned meat as fit meat for consumer, the condemned meat and offals should be stained with colouring agents such as Black PN, Brilliant Black BN (E151, Colour Index 197, No. 28440)
- The best and most cost-effective method of rendering unfit meat and offals is by heat treatment in jacketed vessel and thus, whole sterilization is ensured

9

Muscle and Its Associated Structures

Muscle structure

- All muscles are composed of muscle fibres which are the structural unit of muscles
- In turn, every single muscle fibre is made up of numerous smaller components called myofibrils
- Functional unit of myofibril is sarcomere

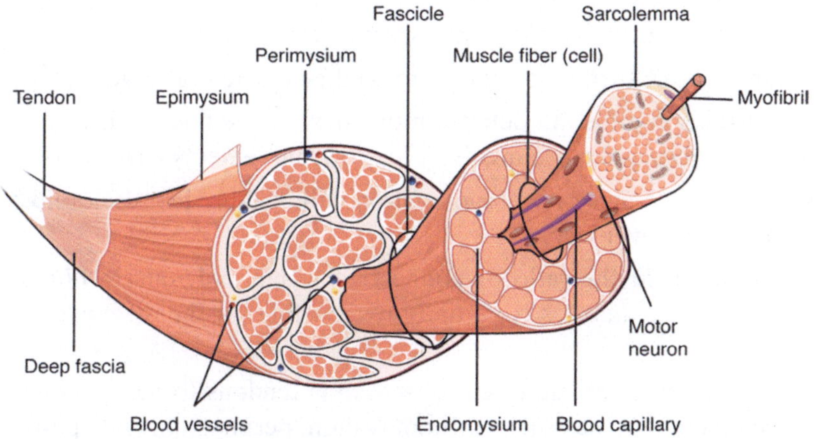

Fig 9.1. Muscle structure (Structure of skeletal muscle. Open Library Anatomy & Physiology. Accessed on 22/02/2025 https://ecampusontario.pressbooks.pub/hhnp4/chapter/10-2-skeletal-muscle/)

Connective tissues associated with muscle

- Whole muscle is surrounded by a sheath of connective tissue called **epimysium**
- Whole muscle is divided into muscle bundles by **perimysium** formed out of connective tissue septa originating from the interior surface of the epimysium separating the muscle fibres
- The perimysium contains the blood vessels and nerves

- Similarly, muscle bundles are divided into single distinct muscle fibre by the **endomysium** formed from the fine connective tissue septa originating from the inner surface of the perimysium
- Thus, connective tissue covering each muscle fibre is called endomysium
    - Epimysium- surrounds the muscle
    - Perimysium- surrounds the muscle fibre bundles
    - Endomysium- surrounds the individual muscle fibre
- Basement membrane is the structure which attaches the collagenous fibres of endomysium with the muscle cell membrane
- Basement membrane is composed of collagen (only 40%) and complex polysaccharides (proteoglycans and glycoproteins)
- Only about 40 per cent of the dry weight of the basement membrane is collagen, the remainder consisting of complex polysaccharides called proteoglycans and glycoproteins
- Sacrcolemma= Basement membrane
- The muscle texture is dependent on the muscle fibre size
- Muscles involved in delicate movements have fine texture *eg.* muscles of the eyes and those involved in gross movements have coarse texture
- However, connective tissue fraction will be more in muscles involved in delicate movements
- Variation in the ratio of connective tissue and muscle fibres among the various muscles is partially responsible for the differences in meat toughness
- Muscle fibres are attached to bones via tendons formed by blending of connective tissues such as endomysium, perimysium and epimysium
- Structure of tendons shows that the collagen fibres found in it have 'crimp' at consistent interval of nearly 100 μm
- This character allows the collagen to bear the early shock of movement by opening the crimps and becoming straightened prior to complete load is borne by the tendon

Connective tissue is made up of

1. Formed elements (Collagen & Elastin) and
2. An amorphous ground substance in which the formed elements are inserted

1. The formed elements are constituted of

i. Collagen fibres-- straight, inextensible and non-branching fibres and

ii. Elastin fibres-- elastic, branching and yellow in colour

Collagen: collagen structure

Primary structure of collagen

- Hydroxyproline makes 12.8% of the peptide chains of collagen of warm-blooded animals
- The collagen is composed of three polypeptide chains which are wound in right hand direction forming helix structure
- Each polypeptide chains of collagen (each chain referred as α chain) has repeating amino-acid sequence consisting of glycine-proline-hydroxyproline- glycine- one of the other amino acids (Fig. 9.2a)
- Collagen is composed of three α chains which are formed by polypeptide chains (Fig. 9.2b)
- One chain (denoted as β-chain) out of the three has a little altered amino acid composition than the other two polypeptide chains (denoted as α1- and α2-)
- There are minimum 12 various forms of collagen each showing a distinct amino acids sequence in its primary structure and linked with diverse carbohydrate molecules
- The three α chains of the collagen arrange themselves in a packed manner assuming helical structure called triple α helix of the tropocollagen (Fig. 9.2c)
- Every third amino acid residue in the α chains of the collagen is glycine and the side chain reveals only hydrogen
- The proline and hydroxyproline content of the polypeptide chain influence the thermal stability of the triple helical structure as well as it affects the eating quality of meat significantly
- The two ends of the α-chains are not involved in the helix formation are referred as N- and C-terminals
- The length of the N- and C-terminals in the α-chains are only 20–25 amino acid
- At all times, the N-terminal region is occupied by lysine amino acid at position 9
- Cysteine is the only amino acid found at the C-terminal end of the type III collagen

- Polypeptide chains are produced by ribosomes and their hydroxylation takes place just before their release in the presence of particular enzymes
- Hydroxylysine amino acid is required to add little quantity of carbohydrate to the collagen
- The enzymes involved need ascorbic acid and oxygen for their action
- Ascorbic acid regulates the conversion of proline into hydroxyproline in the polypeptide chain.
- In case of lack of ascorbic acid, an elastin having low hydroxyproline content is synthesized

Table 9.1: Various types of collagen

Type	Molecular conformation	Presence in different tissues	Hydroxyproline content (residues/1000)	Hydroxylysine content (residues/ 1000)	Glycosylation of hydroxylysine (%)
I	$[\alpha_1 (I)]_2 \alpha_2$	Tendon, bone dentine, dermis, muscle	1	6–8	20
II	$[\alpha_1 (II)]_3$	Cartilage, vitreous humour, intervertebral discs,	2	20-25	50
III	$[\alpha_1 (III)]_3$	Foetal dermis, cardiovascular system, synovial membrane, viscera, muscle	1	6–8	15–20
IV	$\alpha_1 (IV)[\alpha_2 (IV)]_2$	Basement membrane, lens capsule and kidney glomeruli	10	60–70	80
V	$\alpha (V)[\alpha (V)]_2$ and $[\alpha_3 (V)]_3$	Placental membrane, cardiovascular system, lung; minor component of most tissues	2–3	6–8	–

Secondary structure of collagen

- Each of the three α chains of collagen fibre is wound in left-handed fashion to form left handed helix and finally, all the three α chains together wound in such a fashion to form right-handed helical structure—this structure is referred as tropocollagen molecule or collagen protofibril (Fig. 9.2c)
- Tropocollagen molecules self-arrange to produce fibrils and fibrils arrange themselves to produce collagen fibres (Fig. 9.2d)
- The collagen fibres are placed down in a manner forming criss-cross lattice positioned at an angle to the long axis of the muscle

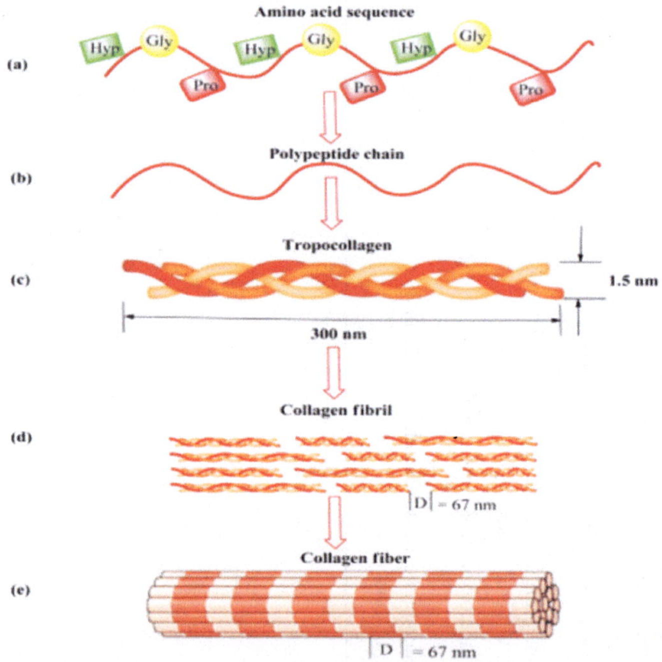

Fig. 9.2. Structure of collagen (Source: Chakraborty, R., Asthana, A., Singh, A. K., Adhikari, R., & Susan, M. A. B. H. (2023). Collagen-a highly developed and abundant fibrous protein: synthesis and characterization. In *Handbook of Natural Polymers, Volume 1* (pp. 489-508). Elsevier Publication)

- Collagen type I, II and III self-aggregate to form fibres whereas collagen type IV is amorphous and are present in the muscle basement membrane along with fibres of other collagen types
- Type V collagen is fibrous and present in the placental membrane however, it is found in minute quantity in many other tissues

- Collagen types VI and VII are filamentous in structure and have little importance in meat
- Only four types of collagen molecule are said to be important for muscle fibres
- Collagen types I and III are present in epimysial, perimysial and endomysial connective tissue, but the epimysium is mainly type I
- Type III collagen is found abundantly in the perimysium
- Endomysium contains equal quantity of types I and III collagen and basement membrane has significant quantity of type IV collagen
- Little quantity of type V collagen are found in the endomysium and the perimysium

The chief post-translational alteration of collagen is the creation of

I. Intramolecular cross- links (between α-chains in the same molecule) and

II. Intermolecular cross- links

  - These cross links (both Intramolecular cross- links & Intermolecular cross- links) are important for imparting great mechanical strength to the collagen. These cross-links are covalent in nature and of three types:
  - *Disulphide bonds*- found in types III and IV collagen as they are the only ones having cysteine amino acid
  - *Divalent bonds*- these bonds combine the α-chains and are produced by the lysine or hydroxylysine aldehydes (reducible in vitro)
  - *More complex bonds*- these bonds combine more than two α-chains and are formed as the collagen matures with age (mature cross-links)

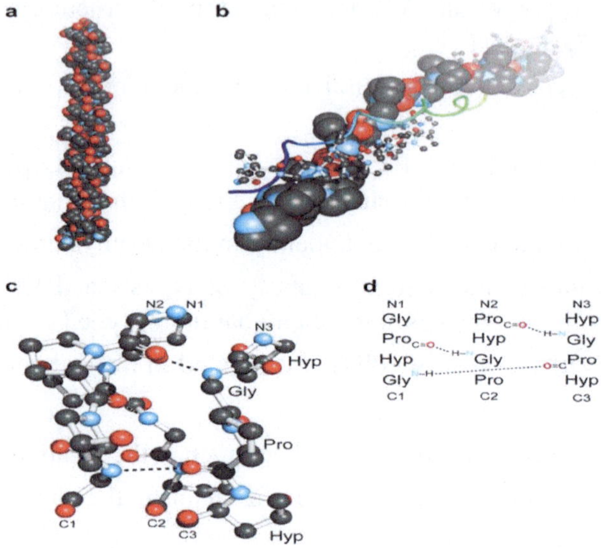

Fig. 9.3. Overview of the triple helix of collagen (a) A collagen triple helix first high-resolution crystal structure, formed using (ProHypGly)4–(ProHypAla)–(ProHypGly)5 [Protein Data Bank (PDB) entry 1cag] (Bella et al., 1994). (b) Visualisation of the image down the axis of a (ProProGly)10 triple helix [PDB entry 1k6f (Berisio et al., 2002)] that has its three strands illustrated in ball-and-stick, space-filling, and ribbon representation. (c) Image of a ball-and-stick representation of a section of a collagen triple helix [PDB entry 1cag (19)], which emphasizes the ladder for the inter strand hydrogen bonds. (d) Stagger image of the three strands found in the segment for panel c (Shoulders and Raines, 2009).

ii. Divalent bonds

- In any tissue, the lysine-derived cross-links depend on the oxidation of aldehydes of particular lysine and hydroxylysine residues (in the non- helical regions at both N- and C- terminal ends of the polypeptide chains) by lysyl oxidase, an enzyme which binds to the nascent collagen fibres (but not to soluble collagen monomers)

$$\begin{matrix}\text{Aldehydes of lysine and} \\ \text{hydroxylysine residues}\end{matrix} \xrightarrow[\text{at non-heical area}]{\text{lysyl oxidase (oxidation)}} \begin{matrix}\text{cross linking of} \\ \text{lysine / hydroxylysine residue}\end{matrix}$$

- The enzyme lysyl oxidase contains copper acting as prosthetic group
- Lack of copper and the administration of β-aminopropionitrile obstruct this oxidation reactions
- Different types of connective tissue diseases are due to failure of any of the biochemical reactions taking place during cross-link formation
- The cross-link formed from two lysine aldehydes is an aldol cross-link and this link can only be intramolecular since it depends on

lysine aldehydes exact opposite location in the two α-chains of the same collagen molecule and the aldol cross-link is found at only at the N-terminal ends

- Aldol cross-links being intramolecular cannot provide the stability to collagen fibres because stability is provided by the intermolecular bonds

Types of Intermolecular bonds formed by lysine aldehydes

I. Aldimine link (dehydro-hydroxy-lysino- norleucine)
II. Oxo-imino link (hydroxylysino-5 oxonorleucine)
III. More complex bonds

I. Aldimine link (dehydro-hydroxy-lysino- norleucine)

- The lysine aldehyde in one α-chain can react with the ε-amino group of the hydroxylysine in the overlapped neighboring molecule of the collagen fibril to form a stable aldimine link called dehydro-hydroxy-lysino-norleucine link
- It is reducible to hydroxy-lysinonorleucine and is heat-labile

$$\text{lysine aldehyde} + \text{hydroxylysine} \xrightarrow{\text{aldimine link formation}} \begin{matrix}\text{dehydro - hydroxy}\\ \text{-lysino - norleucine link}\end{matrix}$$

II. Oxo-imino link (hydroxylysino-5 oxonorleucine)

- A second type of stable cross-link (bond) can be formed between the hydroxylysine aldehyde in the non-helix region of one molecule and the hydroxylysine of a nearby molecule to form a bond which undergoes Amadori rearrangement and becomes an oxo- imino link called hydroxylysino-5 oxonorleucine link

$$\text{hydroxylysine aldehyde} + \text{hydroxylysine} \xrightarrow[\text{Oxo-imino link formation}]{\text{Amadori rearrangement}} \begin{matrix}\text{hydroxylysino - 5 oxonorleucine link}\\ (\text{have oxo - imino bond})\end{matrix}$$

- This bond (cross-link) can be reduced to acid-stable dihydroxy-lysinonorleucine
- Tissues containing small hydroxylated portion of collagen will have enhanced ratios of aldimine to oxoimino intermolecular cross-links and *vice-vera*

III. More complex bonds

- Collagen becomes more and more resistant to disintegration as it matures with the animal age
- This does not happen because of increasing intermolecular bond formation as the number of such bonds decrease with collagen maturation

- Rather, it is due to creation of non-reducible bonds formation between three or more α chains of the collagen and thus, a three-dimensional complex is formed and more tensile strength is generated
- The nature of these mature cross-links is not understood but hydroxyaldohistidine and pyridinoline are the structures liable for development of resistance to breakdown
- Additionally, enhanced glycosylation of lysine residues is also important in the maturation of collagen as the age progresses
- Another responsible factor is the increase in the collagen fibre diameter during maturation with ageing
- The relationship of high meat toughness (as the animal age increases) associated with more number of heat-stable cross-links in muscle collagen cannot explain the observed difference in the meat toughness of different animals of the same age
- Heating collagen at around 65 °C leads to collagen shrinkage with the formation of gelatin and the nature of the cross-links present in the collagen will influence the collagen solubility, the degree of shrinkage and the tension generated during shrinkage
- As the animal age advances, production of more matured and transversed bonds (cross-links) results in development of more tension in collagen on heating
- This tension continues to be high as the heating goes beyond 65 °C in matured animals
- However, in young animals, this collagen tension decreases very much as the temperature of heating rises
- The thermal transition temperature of collagen found in tendon is highly inconsistent and therefore, thermal transition temperature of collagen cannot be used to determine the animal age
- In various goat muscles, as the animal matures with age, there is increase in the shrinkage temperature of intramuscular collagen and this increase is closely related with the increasing pyridinoline content in the collagen
- This pyridinoline is the important end product of the cross-linking pathway comprising hydroxylysine

Elastic fibres

- Elastic fibres—are found in the walls of blood vessels
- They constitutes only small proportion of the muscle connective tissue and on heating, become shrunk and tough thereby, influencing the texture of meat
- In contrary, on heating along with water at more thn 80 °C, collagen fibres become water soluble gelatin
- Major portion of elastin fibre contains an amorphous protein called elastin and the left over portion consists of microfibrillar protein made up of several polar amino acids
- Elastin protein is composed of 40% glycine, 40% hydrophobic amino acids (consisting of 18% valine) and minute quantity of proline and hydroxyproline (1.6%)
- Similar to collagen, cross-links are formed in elastin involving several lysine residues with the help of lysyl oxidase
- In the beginning, like collagen, aldols and aldimines cross-links are formed
- Later, these bonds get condensed to form 1:2- dihydrodesmosine and isodesmosine which are oxidized to form desmosines
- Desmosines are salts of tetramethyl-substituted pyridine and impart fluorescence and yellow colour to elastin
- Once again similar to collagen, with advancing age, elastin turn highly insoluble without formation of additional cross-links
- Tissue macrophages have elastase involved in elastin proteolysis

Types of elastin fibres

1. Coarse elastin fibres
2. Finer elastin fibres

1. Coarse elastin fibres

- Coarse elastin fibres having diameter 5–10 μm are present in the epimysium and perimysium oriented parallel to the long axis of the muscle fibres

2. Finer elastin fibres

- Finer elastin fibres having diameter 1–2 μm are also found in the epimysium and perimysium however, they are positioned at an angle to the axis of muscle fibres and parallel to the network of collagen fibres

- According to the its origin, the structure and arrangement of elastin fibres varies
- Thick elastic fibres are found in greater proportion in the ox ligamentum nuchae and the proteoglycan ground substance separate these fibres
- The elastin fibres found in the blood vessels of arteries and veins are further connected with the collagen fibres and smooth muscle
- In this manner, in association with great number of chondrocyte cells present in connective tissue, elastin fibres of elastic cartilage forms a lace-like network of fibrils

2. Amorphous ground substance

A small part of intramuscular connective tissue are made up of

Proteoglycans

Glycoproteins

Proteoglycans

- Proteoglycans are big molecules having a protein core which is bonded covalently with glycosaminoglycan chains
- Glycosaminoglycan chains-- are repeating disaccharide units of hexosamine and a hexuronic acid related to sulphate esters
- Glycosaminoglycan chains possess high negative charge and so, repel each other resulting in formation of stretched structure which attaches a great amount of water
- The proteoglycans influences the size and orientation of connective tissue fibres and thereby affects the meat texture
- The composition of proteoglycans of various types is presented in Table 9.2

Table 9.2. Composition of different proteoglycans and their location (Bailey and Light, 1989)

Proteoglycan	Disaccharide repeating unit	Location
Chondroitin sulphate	Glucuronic acid and N-acetyl galactosamine	Cartilage: intravertebral disc
Dermatan sulphate	Iduronic acid and N-acetyl galactosamine	Skin: tendon
Heparin sulphate and heparin	(Glucuronic acid and N-acetyl glucosamine + Iduronic acid and N-acetyl glucosamine)	Basement membrane: fibrous tissues
Keratan sulphate	Galactose and N-acetyl glucosamine	Cartilage: cornea: intravertebral disc
Hyaluronic acid	Glucuronic acid and N-acetyl glucosamine	All connective tissue: vitreous body

Glycoproteins

- Glycoproteins (*e.g.* laminin and fibronectin) are also big protein-polysaccharide molecules present in the extracellular matrix
- They anchor cells to basement membranes and other types of collagen

The muscle fibre

- The muscle fibres are the important structural unit of all the muscles
- Muscle fibres are long, narrow, multi- nucleated cells spread throughout the whole length of the muscle and may be of 34 cm length and 10–100 μm in diameter
- Depending on the location, species, breeds and sex, the diameters of muscle fibres fluctuate

Components of skeletal muscle

- A muscle contains muscle fibres of different diameters
- The large diameter fibres are located in the center of the muscle and the small diameter muscle fibres are located at the more peripheral region
- Normally, the muscles containing higher level of pigments have smaller diameter and larger diameter muscle fibres are non- pigmented

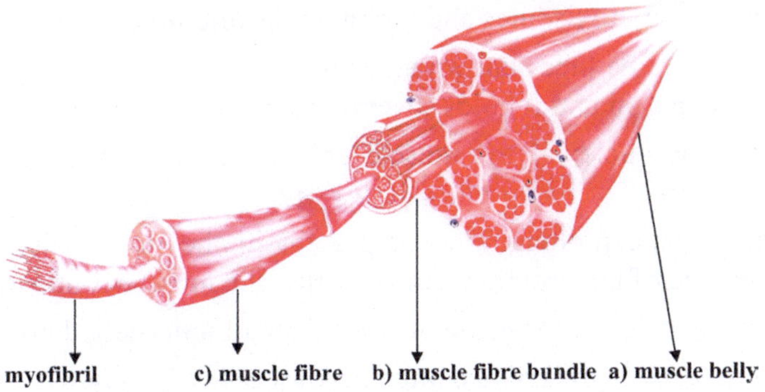

Fig. 9.4. Components of skeletal muscle

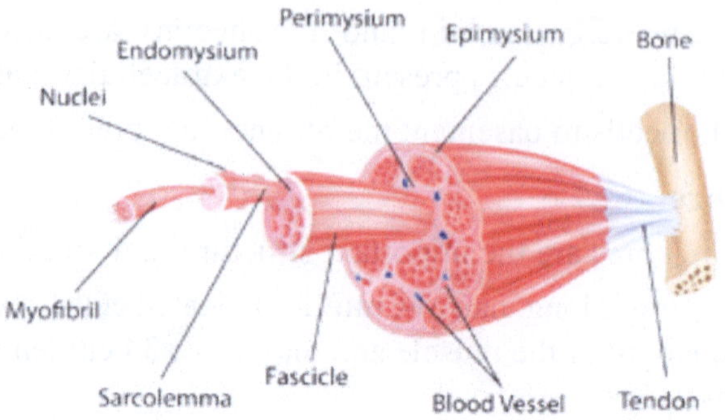

Fig. 9.5. The various muscle components of muscle (*Source:* https://www.gymfailedyou.com/delayed-onset-muscle-soreness/)

- Each muscle fibre is surrounded by a double membrane sheath known as sarcolemma which is present beneath the endomysium connective tissue (Fig. 9.4 & 9.5)
- Within each muscle fibre, there are many myofibrils which are surrounded by a fluid known as sarcoplasm
- The sarcoplasm contains many cellular organelles such as mitochondria, lysosomes, peroxisomes and the sarcoplasmic lipid bodies
- A chain of fine tubes known as sarcotubular system is spread around in the sarcoplasm and it holds several dissolved or suspended materials
- Numerous nuclei of the muscle cell are commonly present near the sarcolemma
- Sarcoplasmic proteins are not present in the myofibrils because the larger size of the protein would obstruct the muscle contraction
- Every muscle fibre is made of several small units called myofibrils
- In turn, each myofibril is composed of the
  - i. Dark or A-band having a central clear zone called the H- zone and
  - ii. Light or I-band having a central dark zone called the Z-line
- The distance between two neighboring Z-lines is the functional unit of the myofibril referred as the sarcomere (Fig. 9.6)
- Each myofibril is composed of several parallel filaments of sarcomere

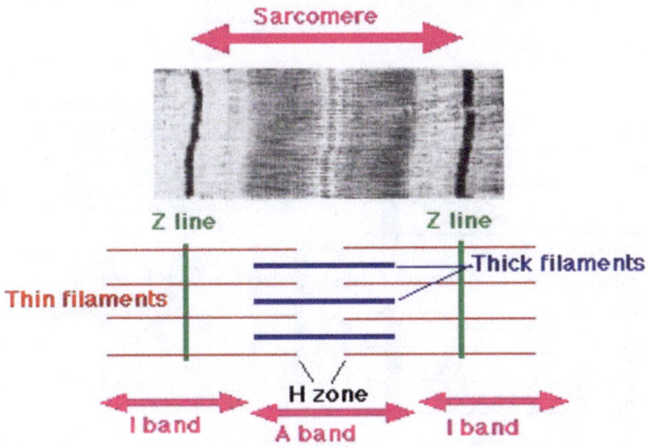

Fig. 9.6. Sarcomere (*Source:* https://commons.wikimedia.org/wiki/File:Sarcomere.gif)

Sarcomeres

- Contractile units of muscle
- Two types of protein myofilaments:
  - Actin: thin filament
  - Myosin: thick filament
- Every myosin filament is encircled by six actin filaments (Fig. 9.7)
- Small contractile myosin bridge are found projecting from each myosin

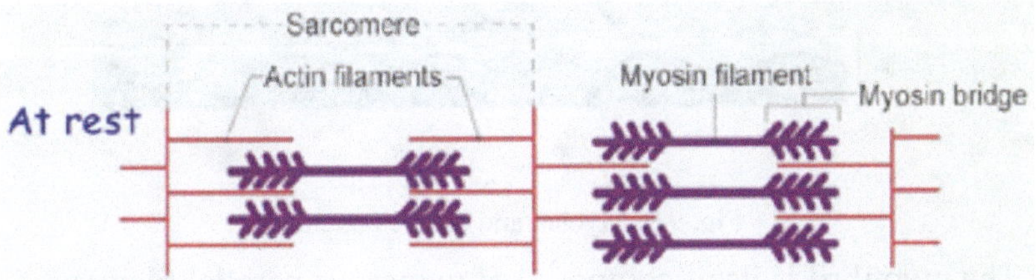

Fig. 9.7. Longitudinal section of myofibril (*Source*: https://slideplayer.com/slide/4452465 /14/ images/15/Longitudinal+section+of+myofibril.jpg)

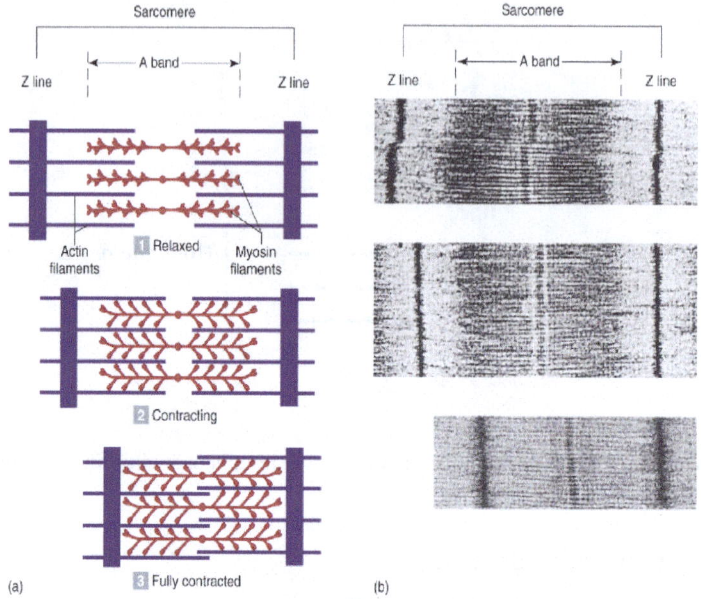

Fig. 9.8. Sarcomere (Howell, S., 2014)

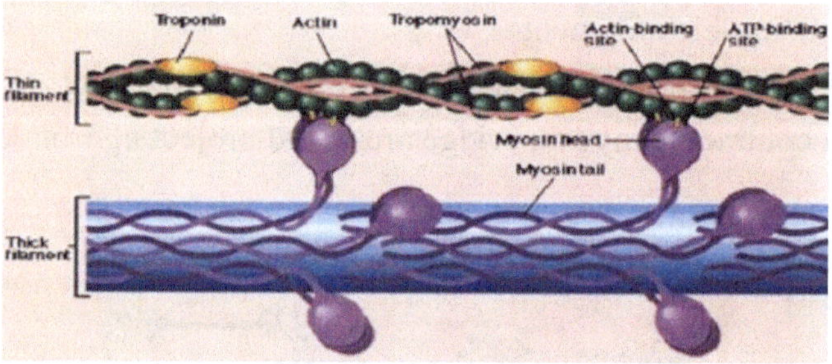

Fig. 9.9. Myosin and actin filaments

- The myofibril is itself composed of numerous parallel filaments
- Few filaments spread out from the *Z*-lines up to the boundary of the *H*-zone and few other filaments extend the whole breadth of the *A*-band
- Those filaments extending through the whole of the A-band are comparatively thick and the filaments which start from the Z-lines and reaches up to the border of the H-zone are comparatively thin (Fig. 9.8 & 9.9)
- The thick and thin filaments represents the contractile proteins known as myosin and actin, respectively

- Every myosin filament is encircled by six actin filaments in hexagonal arrangement
- Between the myosin and actin filaments, tiny projections are found
- The projections are so organized that each sixth one is on the same radial plane of the cylinder of the myosin filament and aligned opposite to one of the six encircling actin filaments

Actin

It consists of

I. F-actin/filamentous actin- made up of G-actin (globular actin)- 2 strands

II. Tropomyosin- 2 strands

III. Troponin- C, T & I (3 in number)

- The actin filaments is composed of two identical chains which are wound to form helical structure containing round sub-units--- known as F-actin/ filamentous actin (Fig. 9.10 & 9.11)
- Two identical chains (strands) of minor myofibrillar protein runs along the each chain/strands of F-actin/ filamentous actin and is referred as tropomyosin
- At every 38.5 nm distance on tropomyosin strands, another protein referred as troponin is present which consists of three sub-units called T, C and I
- Troponin T binds to tropomyosin

Myosin

Myosin consists of 2 monomers of meromyosin

- Each meromyosin monomer is made up of

  I. Head

  II. Short arm &

  III. Tail
- Each myosin molecule looks like tadpole and several myosin molecules aggregate horizontally to form a myosin filament (Fig. 9.11)
- The myosin molecules are so arranged that the 'tails' face towards each other and the 'head' is projected in the direction of Z-lines

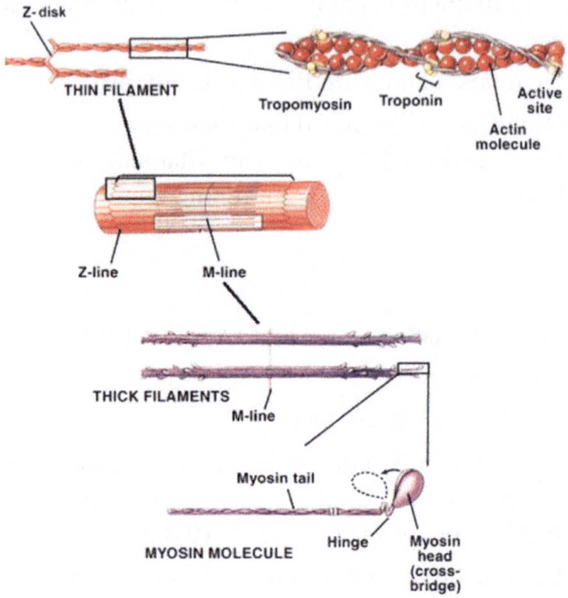

Fig. 9.10. Cross-bridge formation between Actin and myosin

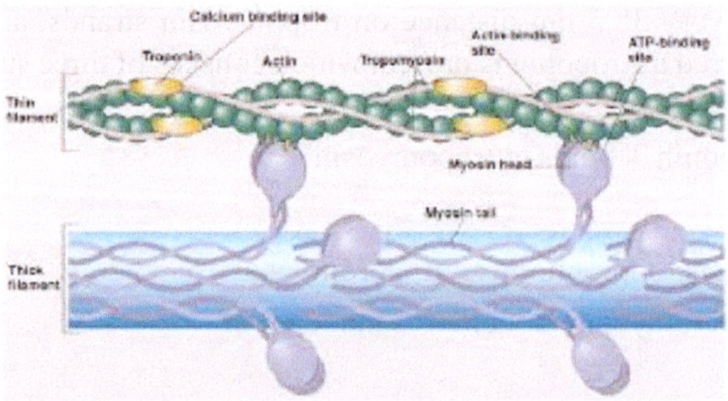

Fig. 9.11. Fine details of actin and myosin filaments

- The aggregation of myosin molecules results in formation of myosin filament having cylindrical body with tapering ends measuring almost 1.5 mm in length
- Thus, a myosin filament is composed of nearly 200 myosin molecules and its length is 1500 Å
- Each molecule is made up of two similar units called meromyosin (Fig. 9.12 & 9.13)
- Each meromyosin has a

i. 'Tail' (light meromyosin)

ii. 'Collar' (heavy meromyosin S–2) and

iii. 'Head' region (heavy meromyosin S-1)

- Use of trypsin to digest myosin results in the release of the heavy and light meromyosin fragments
- Acetylation results in the release of three small fragments of MW 20,000 Da

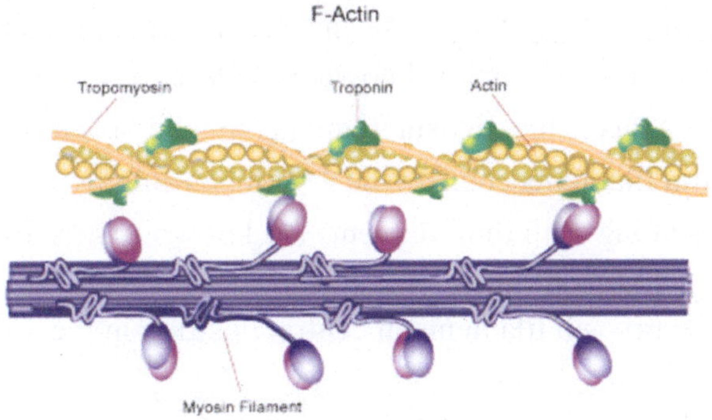

Fig. 9.12. Myosin and actin molecules

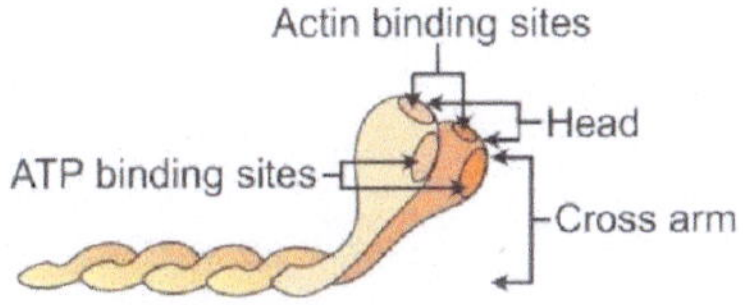

Fig. 9.13. Myosin molecules

- 'Head' region contains three light sub-units
- One of these 3 sub-units have amino acids N^{ε}-methyl lysine and 3-methylhistidine as portion of the myosin molecule
  - In myosin, after peptide bond formation, these two amino acids undergo methylation
  - The intermediate region 'collar' (heavy meromyosin S–2) which is the point of joining of the 'tail' shaft (light meromyosin) and the 'head' (heavy meromyosin S-1) of the myosin molecule is vulnerable to the proteolytic enzymes attack
  - The 'tail' (light meromyosin) of the myosin filaments is oriented as right-wound tertiary coil consisting of three secondary coils and each three secondary coils comprises of three left-wound helical primary strands

- The heavy meromyosin heads of the myosin molecules are regularly disposed along the myosin filament to give nine in the helical repeat distance

Structures present in the M-zone in the center of the myosin filaments

- There are two distinct structures present in the *M*-zone (Fig. 9.14)
  i. *M*-bridge
  ii. Thin filaments
- Perpendicular to the long axis of myosin filaments, 3 to 5 parallel striations are found which is known as *M*-bridge (Fig. 9.16)
- *M*-bridge connects the myosin filaments to their six adjacent neighbours
- In turn, thin filaments connect the *M*-bridges among themselves
- *M*-bridges along with thin filaments are known as *M* substance
- The bridge-filament lattice structure of *M* substance is responsible for holding the myosin filaments in central position in the sarcomere

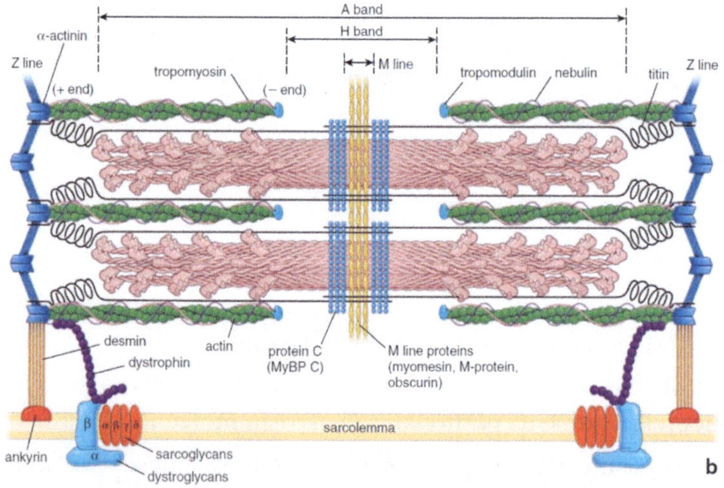

Fig. 9.14. Microscopic view of different molecular structures of a sarcomere. Kindly note the parallel M line proteins in the middle of myosin filaments

Gap-filaments **(Connectin)**

- Referred as 'gap-filaments' because they become visible in the gap developed between the A- and I- bands when both are stretched beyond their overlapping limit
- Observed between the A- and I- bands, it extends from the center of A-band in a sarcomere spreading through the *Z*-line transversing through the I- band and ending at the center of A-band in nearby sarcomere

- Gap-filaments are made up of an elastic protein known as 'connectin'
- Connectin protein extends throughout the length of sarcomere

Connectin (Gap filament proteins) is distinguished into two proteins

i. Titin (10% of myofibrillar proteins)-'T-filaments'
ii. Nebulin (5% of myofibrillar proteins)

Titin (T-Filaments)

- Titin is the main protein of the 'gap filaments' and is also called 'T-filaments' (Fig. 9.14)
- Titin or T-filament is the largest protein (M.W 3000 kDa) present in sarcomere
- The titin/T-filament is composed of single giant molecule which is attached to the thick filament (myosin)
- Six number of T-filaments or titin protein chain are present in every half-sarcomere, originating at the *M*-line and passing through the adjacent *Z*-line and reaches up to *M*-line at the adjoining sarcomere
- Porcine and bovine titin have a comparatively high denaturation temperature of 75.6 and 78.4 °C, respectively
- It controls the particular arrangement of myosin and other filament components of sarcomere

Nebulin

- Nebulin is thin and continuous protein chain transversing from the center of A-band passing through the Z-line and reaching up to the center of next A-band and thus, extending on both sides of a *Z*-line (Fig. 9.15)
- Nebulin binds along the whole length of thin (actin) filament

End structures of actin filament

- The end points of the actin (thin) filaments are 'capped' by three different proteins:

  i. Zeugmatin

  ii. α-actinin and

  iii. Tropomodulin

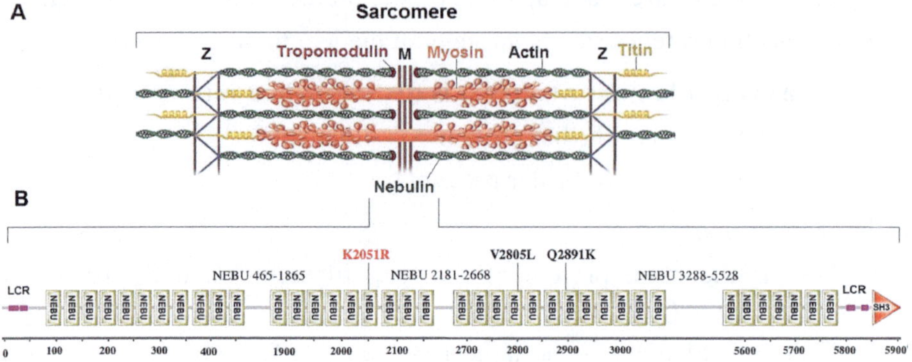

Fig. 9.15. Diagram showing nebulin and tropomodulin

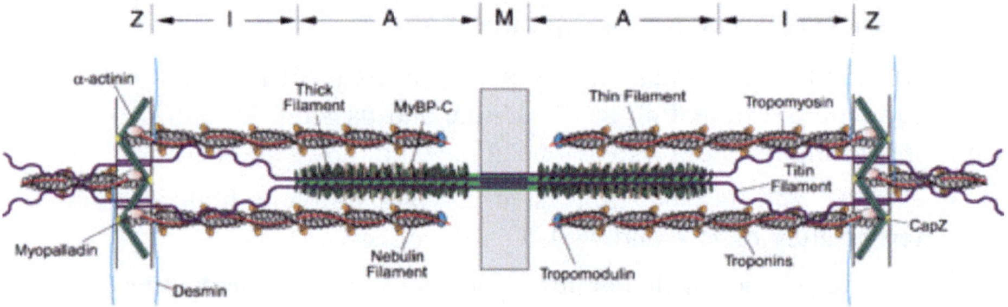

Fig. 9.16. Diagram showing titin filaments, desmin and other structures

- Desmin is a salt-insoluble protein which forms collars within the plane of the *Z*-line preserving the arrangement of neighboring sarcomeres (Fig. 9.16)
- Desmin and connectin ('T-filament' or 'gap-filament' protein) together forms the filamentous cytoskeleton of the muscle fibre apart from the well-known actin and myosin filamentous system (Fig. 9.17)
- Other constituents of the cytoskeleton system are vinculin and talin proteins which keep the actin attached to the cell membrane
- Similar to desmin, vinculin forms a rib-like bands (or costameres) at the *Z*-line around the muscle fibre
- Another protein known as myozenin (calsarcin 2) gets attached to alpha actin and is responsible for controlling the spacing of the actin filaments
- The myofibrillar components interact with the extracellular matrix through the myofibrillar cytoskeleton involving two group of proteins

  i. The dystrophins and

  ii. The integrins

- Integrins are dimeral proteins made up of one α and one β chain with the possibility of minimum 24 combinations of these two chains
- The β chain provides attachment of the cell membrane to the cell body
- The integrin is utmost important in attaching the cell body to the membrane matrix
- Integrin linkage complexes found on the cell surface also hold many signalling proteins such as α-actinin, talin, vinculin and several kinases

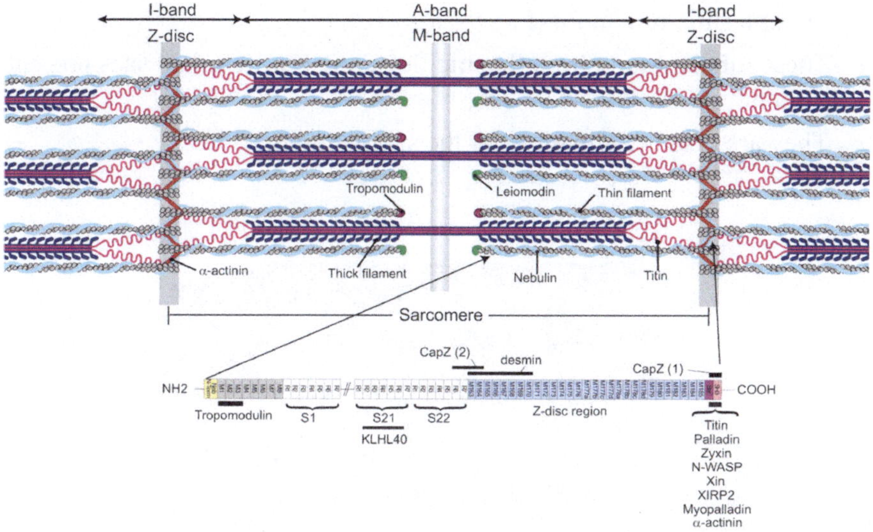

Fig.9.17. The structure of nebulin and the location of its binding partners (Chu *et al.*, 2016).

Organelles of sarcoplasm

- The skeletal mitochondria are present between the myofibrils near the *Z*-line and are particularly present in more number in active muscles
- The peroxisomes found in the sarcoplasm are notable for containing fatty acyl-CoA oxidase and catalase which are involved in production and destruction of H_2O_2, respectively (H_2O_2 formed during the oxidation of fatty acids)
- These organelles are especially numerous in tissues involved in high fat oxidation such as heart muscle and in other tissues
- Peroxisomes are more effective in oxidizing long chain fatty acids (having 20–26 carbon in the long chain) compared to mitochondria
- Every myofibril is encircled by a distinct network known as the sarcotubular system (Fig. 9.18 & 9.19)
- The sarcotubular system consists of two series of tubules:

i. Longitudinal tubules – called 'sarcoplasmic reticulum'

- Spread parallel to the myofibrils and along the sarcomeres, are linked at fixed distances. These tubules join together normally prior to each *Z*-line to form a terminal sac

ii. Transverse tubules- 'T'-system

- Another tubular system running transversely (therefore, called 'T'-system) across the myofibrils originating from the longitudinal sarcoplasmic reticulum (Fig. 9.18)
- These tubules starts from the middle of a pair of terminal sacs present at the adjacent sarcomeres
- They are also invaginations of the sarcolemma

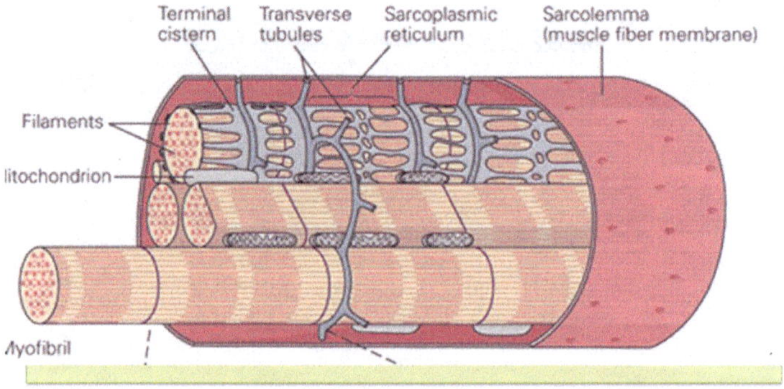

Fig. 9.18. Organelles of sarcoplasm

Sarcotubular system

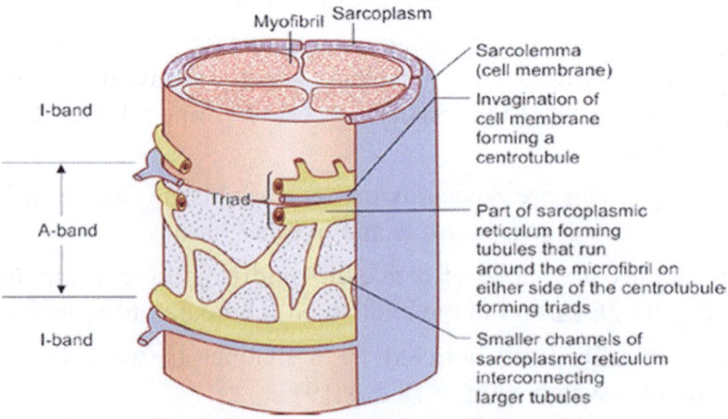

Fig. 9.19a. Sarcotubular system of the muscle cell (longitudinal view)

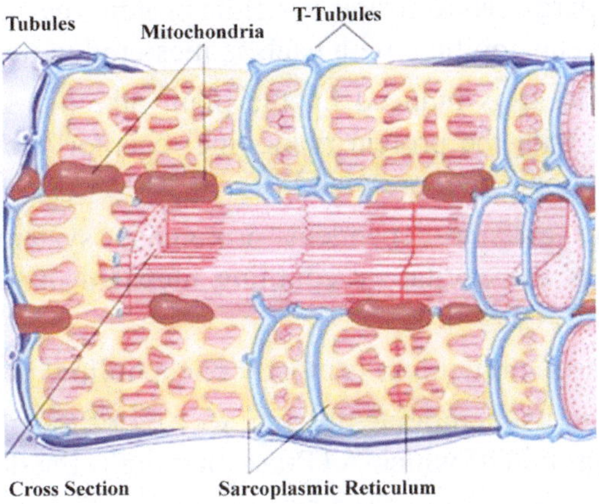

Fig. 9.19b. Sarcotubular system of the muscle cell (cross-sectional view)

- 'Triad', junction between the transverse and the longitudinal tubules on each side, is involved in coupling mechanism
- A big five-unit protein complex known as L-type calcium channels (LTC) is linked with the 'T'-tubules which is the calcium channels of the sarcolemma
- Principally, LTC is involved in many different Ca^{++} ions dependent cellular activities such as commencement of skeletal muscle contraction and is predominantly found in skeletal muscle
- Cyclic AMP-dependent protein kinase is involved in the phosphorylation of the α_1 and β sub-units of LTC which is a precondition for ion passage through the channels
- However, the α_1 sub-unit of LTC is self-reliant to act as an efficient ion channel
- LTC combine with dihydropyridine and forms a receptor called dihydropyridine receptor
- Commencement of muscular contraction is regulated by the degradation by calpains (calcium activated protease) and by the inhibition by calpastatin
- Yet another big protein complex known as junctional foot protein (JFP) situated at the triad junction is projected from the sarcoplasmic reticulum (longitudinal tubules) membrane
- Initially, during muscular contraction the excitatory impulse from the depolarized sarcolemma is conveyed by the 'T' tubules to the sarcoplasmic reticulum which releases Ca^{++} ions

- Ca^{++} ions undergo sequestering by acidic proteins calsequestrin and thus, 40 Ca^{++} ions can combine with each sequestered molecule
- Ca^{++} ions release is induced by the plant alkaloid such as ryanodine which binds with the protein ryanodine receptor possessing similarity with the junctional foot protein (JFP)
- Usually, the calcium-dependent proteinase system is efficient in interacting by the excitatory coupling mechanism of muscle through both LTC and JFP
- The sarcoplasmic reticulum is mostly phospholipid in nature
- It possesses in its membrane nearly 1 to 10% of the phospholid content as intrinsic protein of which ATP-ase enzyme is the dominant one
- On relaxation, the membrane of sarcoplasmic reticulum pumps Ca^{++} ions from the cell interior of cell into the sarcoplasmic reticulum tubular system

Recommended videos

https://www.youtube.com/watch?v=oTo4xNMEmfc

https://www.youtube.com/watch?v=d1eXGmrXEJY&t=4s

References

Bella, J., Eaton, M., Brodsky, B., & Berman, H. M. (1994). Crystal and molecular structure of a collagen-like peptide at 1.9 angstrom resolution. Science, 266(5182), 75-82.

Berisio, R., Vitagliano, L., Mazzarella, L., & Zagari, A. (2002). Crystal structure of the collagen triple helix model [(Pro-Pro-Gly) 10] 3. Protein Science, 11(2), 262-270.

Chu, M., Gregorio, C. C., & Pappas, C. T. (2016). Nebulin, a multi-functional giant. Journal of Experimental Biology, 219(2), 146-152.

Howell, S. (2014). A Unified Theory of Human Skeletal Muscle Growth and Application to Resistance Training. International Journal of Sciences: Basic and Applied Research (IJSBAR)(2014) Volume 9, No 1, pp 1-79.

Shoulders, M. D., & Raines, R. T. (2009). Collagen structure and stability. Annual Review of Biochemistry, 78, 929-958.

10

Molecular Basis of Muscle Contraction and Relaxation

Introduction

- Arrival of the nerve stimulus at the motor end plate result in reversal of the polarization of the sarcolemmal surfaces and the muscle gets activated
- This causes momentarily loss of potassium and sodium ions impermeability by the sarcolemma and Ca^{++} ions combined with calsequestrin in the sarcotubular system gets dissociated bringing Ca^{++} ion equilibrium with the sarcoplasm
- The junctional foot protein (JFP) and the L-type calcium channel (LTC) are the two big protein complexes responsible for the calcium release mechanism (Fig. 10.1)
- This leads to increase in level of Ca^{++} ion from nearly 0.10 mM to 10 mM
- Thus, troponin C, the calcium-binding site of the troponin complex becomes saturated bringing a structural modification resulting in interaction of actin with the $MgATP^{2-}$ on the *H*-meromyosin heads of the myosin molecule as the troponin I, the inhibitory protein, no more inhibits this interaction
- The interaction of actin with the $MgATP^{2-}$ intensely activate contractile ATP-ase near the bonding leading to break down of $MgATP^{2-}$ to $MgADP^{-}$ at a greater rate and liberating energy for inward (towards the sarcomere center) pulling of the actin filament
- This leads to breaking of bond between actin and myosin and thus, the myofibrillar part involved in above mentioned activity gets contracted
- The $MgADP^{-}$ on myosin is recharged to $MgATP^{2-}$ by direct exchange with cytoplasmic ATP by the action of :

  a) ATP: creatine phospho- transferase or

  b) ATP: AMP phosphotransferase

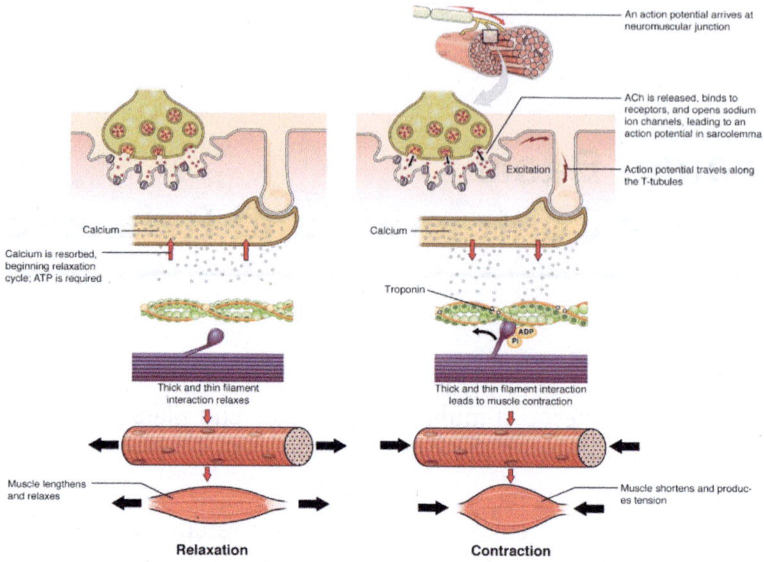

Fig. 10.1. Diagram showing muscle contraction and relaxation through cross-bridge cycling

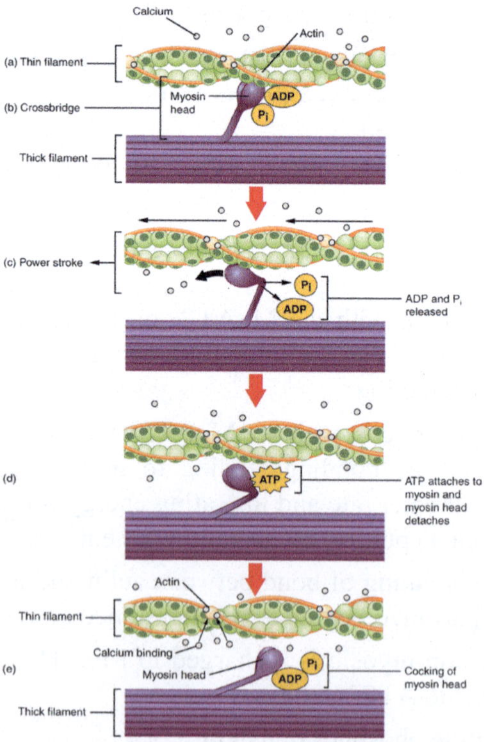

Fig.10.2. Diagram showing muscle contraction and relaxation

- This process continues repetitively till surplus of Ca^{++} ions saturates troponin C and myosin cross-bridges bonding with the myosin-binding sites on actin at successively peripheral locations as the interdigitation continues
- Interdigitation of the actin and myosin filaments may include tilting movements of the cross-bridges formed between the S-1 subunit of myosin and the actin

Binding of myosin cross-bridges with the myosin-binding sites on actin

- $MgATP^{2-}$ is attached to the *H*-meromyosin cross-bridge via a polypeptide chain
- At rest, the polypeptide chain helices are stretched out by mutual repulsion produced by the negative charge on $MgATP^{2-}$ at one end and a net negative charge at the another end (having the polypeptide chain linked to the *H*- meromyosin)
- In this manner, the myosin cross-bridges are capable to join with the myosin-binding sites on actin

Role of Ca^{2+} ions in muscle contraction

- Once muscle is stimulated, Ca^{++} ions negate the negative charge on $MgATP^{2-}$ and thus, eradicate the repulsive action on the coils of the polypeptide chain (Fig. 10.3)
- This cause the polypeptide chain to adopt the α-helix structure and to bind with the actin
- Linking with the actin allows dragging the actin inwards up to a distance equal to the distance of spacing between the two consecutive myosin-binding sites on actin
- On the $MgADP^{2-}$ being recharged to $MgATP^{2-}$, the polypeptide chain gets re-extended
- When the muscle contraction stimulus stops, Ca^{++} ions are reabsorbed by the sarcoplasmic reticulum pump into the sarcotubular system and Ca^{++} ions level reaches to the rest level of 0.10 mM and the required energy for reabsorption is provided by the ATP
- The sarcoplasmic reticulum possesses little ATP-ase activity
- ATP is also required to reestablish the differential distribution of Na^{+} ions between the two surfaces of the sarcolemma which is involved in generating the action potential on nerve stimulation

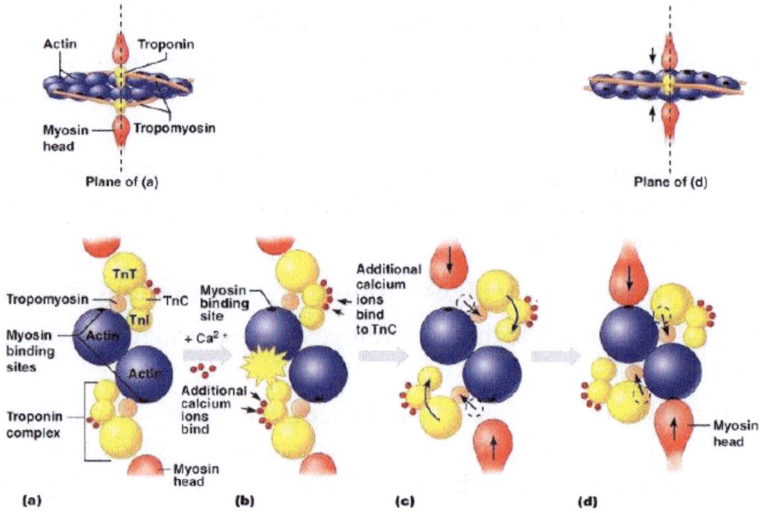

Fig.10.3. Role of Ca^{2+} in muscle contraction

- Once Ca^{++} ions saturation is lost, resting configurations are adopted by troponin C and troponin I whereas troponin I inhibits the interaction between myosin and actin
- The gap filaments possessing certain elasticity, support in pulling the actin filaments towards the outside from their interdigitation with those of myosin so that the resting length of the sarcomere is restored
- Higher concentration of Ca^{++} ions in the sarcoplasm not only initiates the interaction between actin and myosin bringing muscular contraction but higher level of Ca^{++} ions also activates:
  - Myosin light chain kinase (involved in phosphorylation of one of the light chain components of myosin) and
  - Phosphorylase *b* kinase (involved in phosphorylation of troponins T and I).
- Troponin needs the attachment of tropomyosin for its preventive action on actomyosin ATP-ase
- Muscle contraction takes place only when there is system making available the sufficient ATP supply
- Sarcoplasmic proteins, the insoluble as well as soluble, have crucial part in the supply of ATP
- ATP is synthesized again from ADP and creatine phosphate (CP) in the presence of creatine kinase enzyme which is one of the soluble proteins of the sarcoplasm:

ADP + CP → creatine + ATP

- In living animal, resynthesis of ATP from ADP by respiration is the principal source of ATP in which muscle glycogen (or sometimes fatty acids) is broken down into carbon dioxide and water
- The sarcoplasm also contains muscle pigment known as myoglobin which is very different from the haemoglobin pigment of the blood
- Haemoglobin functions as a temporary oxygen storage site in muscle
- The enzymes involved in respiration are oxygen-consuming enzymes especially the cytochrome system and other enzymes needed for ATP production and transformation of pyruvic acid to carbon dioxide and water are found in the insoluble particles called the mitochondria
- Mitochondria is distributed in the sarcoplasm
- Several of the glycolytic and respiratory enzymes need vitamins or trace metals as co-factors: and the muscle composition reveals this requirement

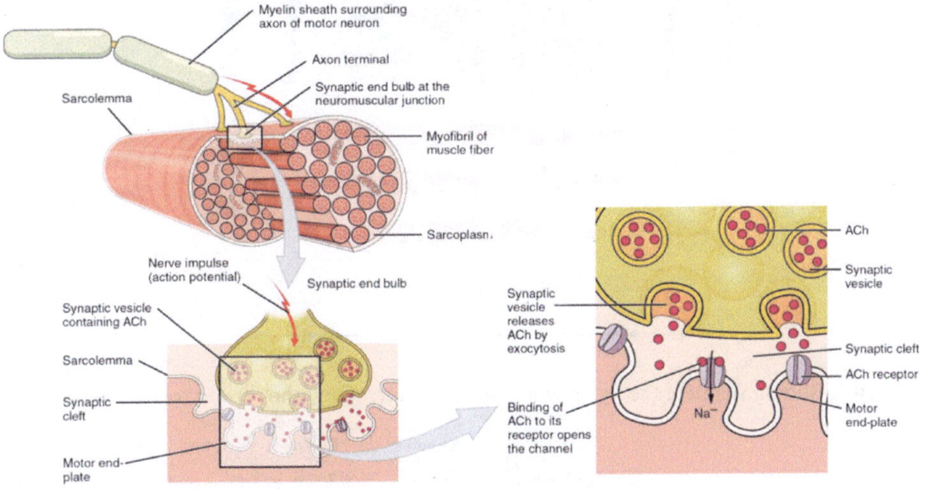

Fig.10.4. Motor end-plate and innervation

Role of calcium (Ca^{+}) in muscle contraction

1. Stimulates neurotransmitter release
2. Activates Ca^{+} release from SR
3. Stimulates sliding of myofilaments and ATPase activity
4. Triggers glycogen breakdown & ATP synthesis

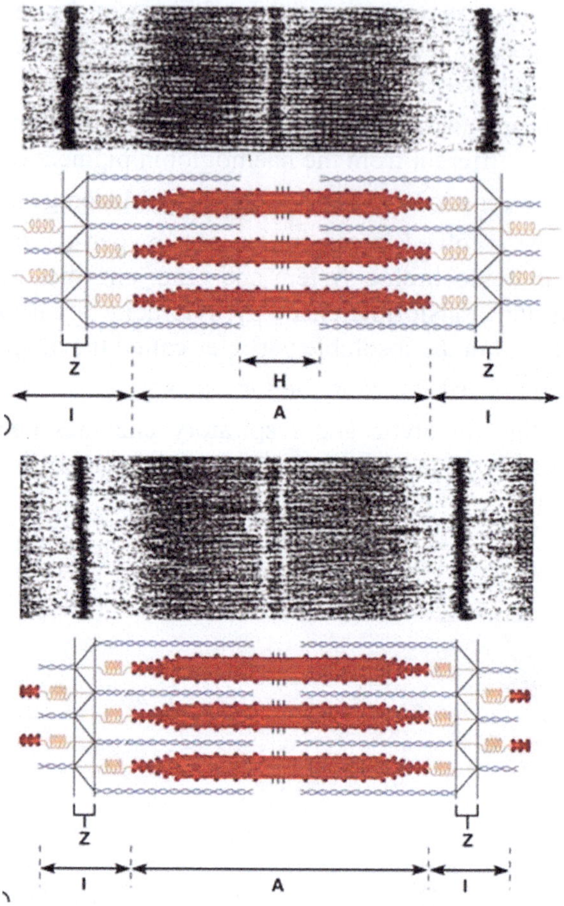

Fig. 10.5. Sliding filament theory showing muscle contraction (above) and relaxation (below)

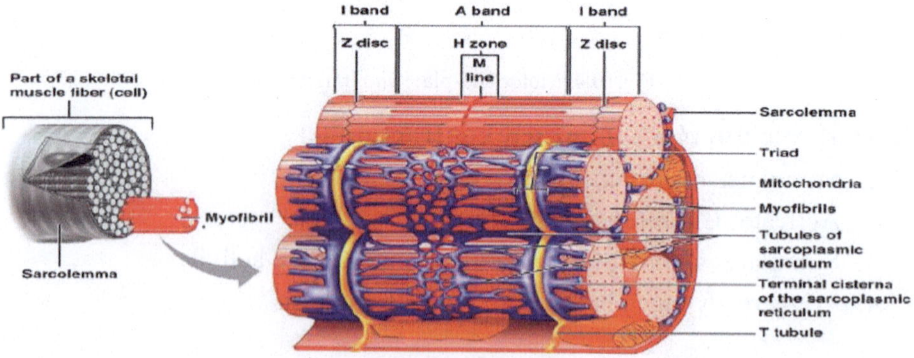

Fig. 10.6. Figure showing muscle fibres being surrounded by sarcoplasmic reticulum and other microscopic structures

Sliding Filament Theory

1. All of the myofibrils contracts together by the movement of the insertion towards the origin of the muscle (Fig. 10.5)
2. Contraction of the sarcomere causes the contraction/shortening of the myofibrils (The distance between Z lines is reduced)
3. Shortening of the sarcomere is characterized by no change in the length of actin and myosin filaments
4. Sliding is accomplished by the powerful pulling of the actin by the myosin cross bridges over the myosin filaments
5. The length of the A band does not change during the contraction but the Z-lines are pulled toward the centre of the A band
6. Neighbouring A bands are drawn nearer to each other and the lengths of I bands between them become shortened
7. The length of H-band shortens during contraction as the thin actin filaments are drawn towards the centre of the H-band

Main events occurring during contraction of muscle

1. The distal end of a motor neuron produces acetylcholine (Fig. 10.7 & 10.8)
2. Acetylcholine diffuses through the gap at the neuromuscular junction
3. This stimulates the sarcolemma and a muscle impulse moves over the surface of the muscle fibre and via the transverse tubules, reaches the deeper part of muscle fibre and finally arrives at the sarcoplasmic reticulum
4. Ca^{2+} ions diffuse into the sarcoplasm from the sarcoplasmic reticulum and combine with troponin molecules
5. Tropomyosin molecules move and uncover particular sites on actin filament
6. Actin and myosin filaments form bonding called myosin cross–bridges
7. Actin filaments are drawn inward by myosin cross–bridges
8. This results in muscle fibre shortening and muscle contraction takes place

Main events occurring during relaxation of muscle

1. Enzyme acetylcholinestrase break downs acetylcholine and thus, the muscle membrane does not gets stimulated any more

2. Ca^{2+} ions are vigorously transported into the sarcoplasmic reticulum
3. The bridge between the actin and myosin filaments are broken down by ATP resulting in re-opening of cross–bridges
4. Troponin and tropomysin molecules prohibit the linkage formation between myosin and actin filaments
5. Thus, muscle fibre becomes relaxed but remains prepared till the arrival of next stimuli

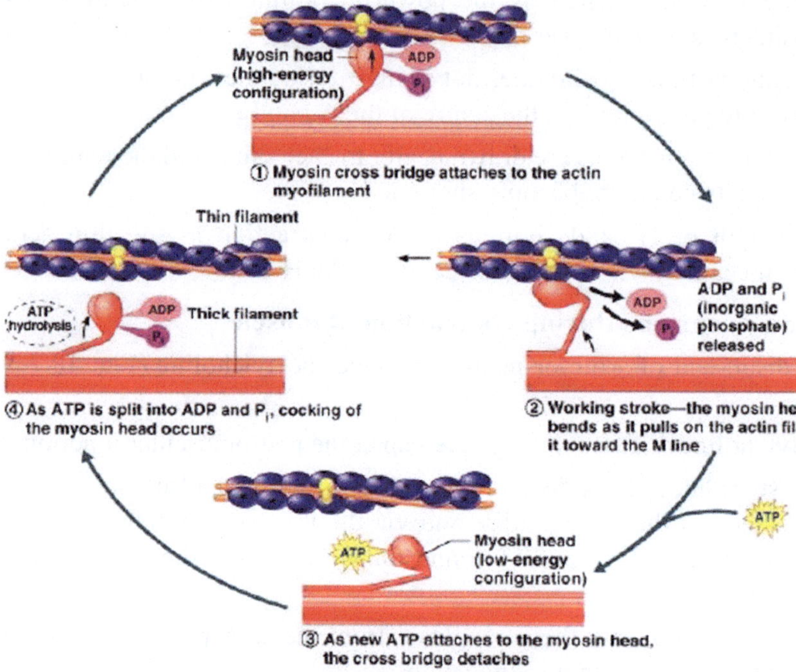

Fig. 10.7. Sliding of actin over myosin

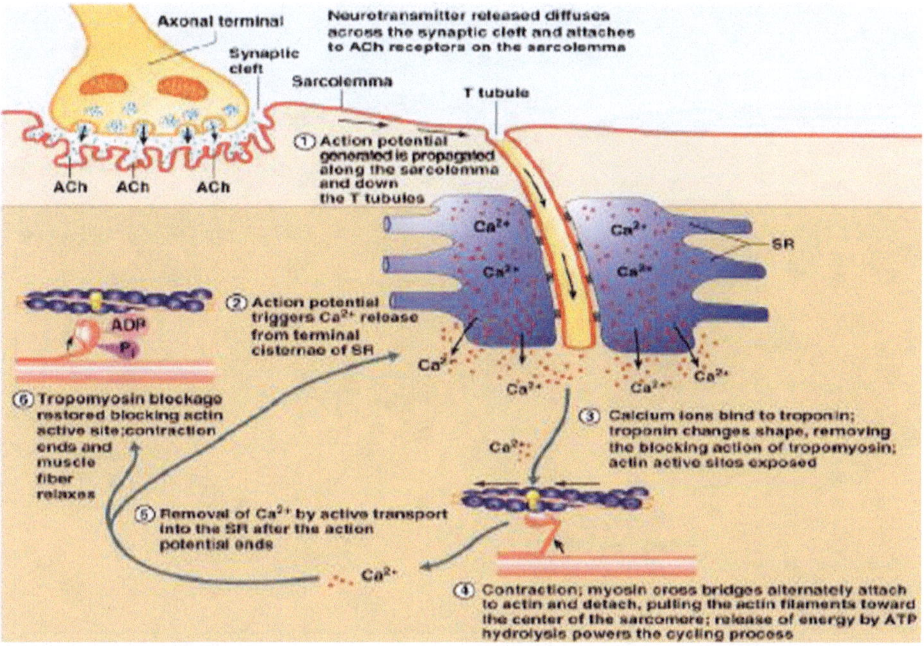

Fig.10.8. Role of neurotransmitters and subsequent Ca^{2+} ions release in muscle contraction

11

Molecular Composition of Muscle Proteins

Constituents of meat

i. Water- 75%
ii. Protein- 19%
iii. Soluble and non-protein substances- 3.5%
iv. Fat- 2.5%

- The muscle fibre is important unit of muscular tissue consisting of
  a) Myofibrils- formed protein structures embedded in sarcoplasmic fluid
  b) Sarcoplasmic reticulum- a fine system of tubules
  c) Sarcolemma- a very thin membrane surrounding the myofibrils and around the exterior side of this membrane, the connective tissue is found
- 19% of protein in the muscle is muscle fibre (Table 11.1)
- α-alanine, glycine, glutamic acid and histidine are the major free amino acids present in the fresh muscle

Muscle proteins

The muscle proteins can be roughly classified into:

1. Sarcoplasmic proteins- Water Soluble Proteins- proteins soluble in water/dilute salt
2. Myofibrillar proteins- Salt Soluble Proteins- proteins soluble in concentrated salt solutions
3. Insoluble proteins- Not soluble in concentrated salt solutions- the connective tissue and other structural proteins

1. Sarcoplasmic proteins

- Many of these proteins are enzymes involved in glycolytic pathway and might be found in more than one form (isozymes)

- Hence, most of the sarcoplasmic proteins are distinguished as glycolytic enzymes
- The glycolytic enzymes are the main constituents of the sarcoplasmic proteins and are attached to the actin filaments (myofibrillar protein)
- This attachment provides them better regulation over the enzymatic bioreactions in the muscle

Table 11.1: Chemical composition of muscle after rigor mortis but prior to putrefactive post-mortem changes

S. No.	Components of muscle	% weight on wet weight basis
1.	Water	75
2.	Protein—divided into 3 categories	19
	i) Myofibrillar protein (myosin (5.5%), actin (2.5%), connectin, nebulin, tropomyosin, troponins *etc.*)	11.5
	ii) Sarcoplasmic protein (creatine kinase, aldolase, myoglobin, haemoglobin, other glycolytic enzymes *etc.*)	5.5
	iii) Connective tissue & organelles (collagen, elastin, mitochondrial *etc.*)	2.0
3.	Lipid	2.5
4.	Carbohydrate (lactic acid, glycogen, glucose *etc.*)	1.2
5.	Miscellaneous soluble non-protein substances (nitrogenous creatinine (1.65%), inosine monophosphate)	2.3

- On electrical stimulation, the amount of bound (attached) glycolytic enzymes enhances and thereby stimulating the glycolysis and reduces as the electrical stimulation ends
- In every helical repeat of the F-actin, 14 units of G-actin are present
- Two binding sites are present in each helical repeat of the F-actin
- Out of these two sites, triose phosphate dehydrogenase favorably cover one site but aldolase can cover both the sites
- Few glycolytic enzymes do not bind to F-actin enzymes but binds with the enzymes which are already combined with triose phosphate dehydrogenase
- Thus, triose phosphate isomerase binds to both aldolase and triose phosphate dehydrogenase which are already bound to F-actin
- It is remarkable to realize that these enzymes are organized spatially in their accurate sequence in the glycolytic pathway
- In this way, many enzymes groups create distinct metabolic compartments from which the metabolites are conveyed from the

enzymes which produce them to those enzymes which act on them ('metabolic channelling')

- Glycogen has two sites for phosphorylase binding
- Besides binding at F-actin, the glycolytic enzymes bind to other sites in the muscle fibres such as the sarcolemma, the sarcoplasmic reticulum and the membranes of the nuclei and mitochondria
- Phosphorylase b seems to be bound at the Z-disk as well as the M-line
- Additionally, creatine kinase is also bound to the M-line

2. Myofibrillar proteins

a) Myosin

- Myosin is the most abundant of the myofibrillar proteins
- The molecule of myosin (MW 500 kDa) is arranged in greatly irregular manner (Fig. 11.1)
- The length to diameter ratio of myosin molecule is nearly 100:1
- It is highly charged molecule owing to rich quantity of dibasic amino acids like glutamic and aspartic acids
- Possesses high affinity for Ca^{++} and Mg^{++} ions
- Myosin is made up of two heavy polypeptide chains and four light polypeptide chains
- Protein degradation splits the myosin into two fragments known as heavy meromyosin (HMM) and light meromyosin (LMM)
- LMM comprises of parts of the two heavy chains
- HMM contains parts of the two heavy chains and the four light chains
- H-meromyosin known for holding all the ATP-ase and actin-binding qualities of myosin, is located on the boundary of the myosin filaments

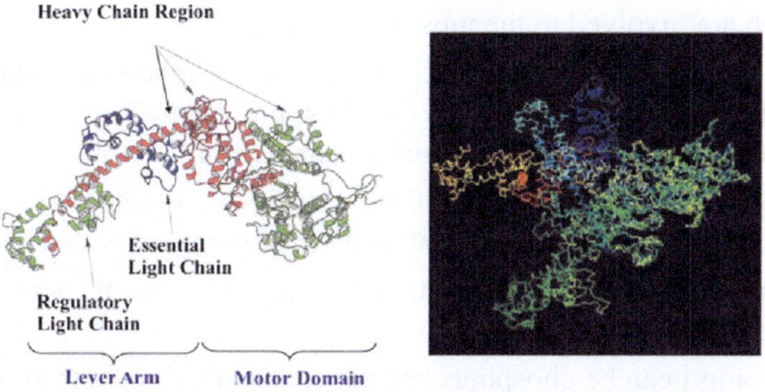

Fig. 11.1. Three dimensional structure of myosin molecules

b) Tropomyosin

- Amino acid composition of tropomyosin and myosin is identical
- Tropomyosin provides a network for attachment of actin filaments with the Z-line and it winds around the whole distance of helical structure of the actin filament

c) Vinulin & integrin

- Vinulin is lipid-binding protein through which the actin filaments are linked to the Z-line and the interior surface of plasma membrane
- Integrin is a complex protein through which the muscle cell proteins of non-specific locations are attached to the muscle cell membrane

d) Actin

- Actin is another main protein of the myofibril
- It can be present in two forms:
  - G-actin of MW around 42 kDa consisting of comparatively small globular units and
  - F-actin- end to end aggregation of G-actin globular units resulting in formation of double chain
- With the help of salts and little quantity of ATP, G-actin polymerizes to form F-actin
- Actually, the contractile actomyosin of active/pre-rigor muscle or the inextensible actomyosin of the muscle during rigor mortis state is formed by the bonding of F-actin with myosin

Other myofibrillar proteins

i. Troponin

- Troponin consists of three major elements known as troponin C, I and T which are involved in the muscle contraction
- The troponin complex encourages the tropomyosin aggregation, combines with calcium and inhibits the formation of actomyosin; α-actinin supports the horizontal attachment of F-actin
- Troponin C having MW 18,000 Da and 159 amino acids has four binding sites for Ca^{++} ions and forms an equimolar complex with troponon I
- Troponin I having MW 21,000 Da and 179 amino acids, prevents actomyosin ATPase
- Troponin I can be phosphorylated at serine and threonine amino acid

- Troponin T having MW 30,000 Da and 259 amino acids combines with tropomyosin and troponin C and phosphorylase b is only enzyme responsible for its phosphorylation

ii. M-line proteins

- Two proteins are present at the M-line:
  i. Myomesin- encourages the horizontal polymerization of only L-meromyosin and not of H-meromyosin. It may combine creatine kinase to the M-line
  ii. Creatine kinase- is the major constituent of the M-bridge
- M-line proteins are necessary for regulating the polarity of the myosin filamenst in the half part of the sarcomere
- Myosin molecule is composed of two shafts (light meromyosin) and a two heads (heavy meromyosin) and two light chain molecules are attached with the each head of the myosin molecule

iii. Additional proteins

- Desmin is the yet another protein located near the Z-line
- Additional proteins which form the Z- line network are μ-actinin, filamin, synemin, vimentin and zeugmatin
- Other insignificant proteins of the myofibrillar protein consists of
  - F- protein – binds with myosin
  - I-protein – in the absence of Ca^{++} ions, prevents the Mg-activated ATP-ase of actomyosin and
  - Para- tropomyosin
- Connectin (also called as 'gap filament'or T-filament) is made up of titin and nebulin
- Desmin and connectin (titin and nebulin) together with vinculin and talin forms the filamentous cytoskeleton network of the muscle fibre

Smooth muscle: few points

- The ratio of myosin (thick) to actin (thin) filaments in skeletal muscle is 1: 2 whereas this ration differs in smooth muscle from 1 : 5 to 1 : 25 based on different types of tissues in which it is present
- Instead of troponin C, calmodulins is present in smooth muscles having characters same as troponin C
- Practically all of the Ca^{++}-binding protein of smooth muscle is of calmodulins type

- Trimethyllysine is an uncommon amino acid found minute quantity in smooth muscles

Amino acid contents of muscle proteins

- Actin, the actinins, troponin C and H-meromyosin have greater proportion of aromatic amino acids compared to their proportion in other structural proteins of muscle fibres
- Actin and the actinins also have comparatively greater proportion of proline
- The MW of troponins C, I and T are 19,500, 23,300 and 40,400 daltons, respectively

12

Post-mortem Glycolysis (Anaerobic Glycolysis)

Post-mortem glycolysis (anaerobic glycolysis)

- Post-mortem glycolysis is the basic function of muscle
- Irreversible anaerobic glycolysis starts after the animal has died and oxygen supply to the muscles is cut
- The various biochemical steps that occur in living animals for the conversion of glycogen into lactic acid when the oxygen supply is insufficient, are basically similar in slaughtered animal also
- After slaughter, during anaerobic glycolysis in normal animals (not in the animals that are exhausted, excited or excessively exercised just prior to slaughter), the glycogen reserve of the muscle decreases appreciably resulting in the lactic acid production which will proceed to a pH level at which the enzymes involved in glycolysis become inactivated
- In classic mammalian muscles this pH will be near to 5.4–5.5 (called Ultimate pH)
- Muscle having almost 600 mg glycogen/100 g muscle at the time of slaughter will reach this pH
- A protein called glycogenin is responsible for starting the glycogenesis (glycogen synthesis) in muscle and it binds with eight glucose molecules to produce a glycosyl-protein (Fig. 12.1)
- Glycosyl-protein is used as primer by the enzyme proglycogen synthase and thus, proglycogen is formed
- This proglycogen is converted into bigger macromolecule by the macroglycogen synthase and its branching enzyme
- Accordingly, for glycogen storage in muscle, presence of glycogenin is the main limiting factor
- When animal undergoes aerobic stress, macroglycogen is specially utilized and in case of anaerobic stress and postmortem glycolysis, proglycogen is metabolized

- Pigs which are the RN- gene carrier, stores greater quantity of glycogen in the muscles in the form of macroglycogen
- Practically, production of lactic acid is single reason for reduction in muscle pH during post-mortem glycolysis
- The final muscle pH achieved is known as the ultimate pH

Glycogenesis (glycogen synthesis)

↓ initiated by

glycogenin (a protein)- major limiting factor for glycogenesis

↓ combines with 8 glucose mol

glycosyl-protein

↓ proglycogen synthase

proglycogen (used during anaerobic stress & post-mortem stress)

↓ macroglycogen synthase

Macroglycogen (used during aerobic stress)

Fig. 12.1. Flowchart of glycogenesis

- Ultimate pH and the isoelectric point of several muscle proteins (also myofibrillar proteins) are same (5.5) and hence, the water holding capacity (WHC) of the muscle will be lower compared to muscle *in-vivo* inspite of absence of muscle denaturation
- At isoelectric point, the muscle electrical impedance is low which is observed at the usual ultimate pH (5.5) but if the ultimate pH remain high (≥6), muscle will show high electrical resistance
- Species, muscle type and inconsistency between animals are some of the intrinsic factors responsible for controlling the rate and the extent of the post-mortem pH reduction
- Similarly, administration of drugs, pre-slaughter and the environmental temperature are some of the extrinsic factors influencing the rate and the extent of the post-mortem pH reduction
- There is big difference in the time duration taken by various pigs in reaching ultimate pH of 5.5 from an initial pH of 7.2 at 37 °C
- Similar variations have been noted between particular muscles of different large ruminants at a specific temperature
- I/V Injection of magnesium sulphate prior to slaughter will reduce the post-mortem glycolysis rate

- I/V administration of calcium salts, adrenaline and noradrenaline will hasten the rate
- I/V administration of adrenaline and tuberculin and insulin shock will cause decreased glycogen content resulting in high ultimate pH
- Post-mortem glycolysis rate enhances with increase in outside temperature above ambient
- The rate of post-mortem glycolysis will tend to be higher in muscles which are slow to cool; and vice versa
- Muscles taking more time to cool will show higher post-mortem glycolysis rate and *vice-versa*

PSE (Pale, soft and exudative meat)

- In this condition, rate of reduction of muscle pH is very high after slaughter in pigs prone to PSE resulting in pH fall to near 5.4 within 40 min of slaughter
- During post-mortem or instantly prior to slaughter, the pig body temperature becomes abnormally high
- PSE affected/prone pigs have shown high Ca^{++} ions levels in the muscles post- mortem
- This will stimulate the ATP-ase of actomyosin and thus, hasten post-mortem glycolysis rate
- The pH falling rate is unusually high even at normal temperature in few pigs and the pH reduction may go on to extraordinarily low ultimate pH of 4.7
- Different diseases affecting the glycogen storage are identified in which particular muscle enzymes are lacking leading to PSE prone pigs
- PSE condition is inheritable in which gene regulated enzymes involved in glycolysis becomes surplus or unbalanced besides structural modifications in the protein complexes such as LTC and JFP related with Ca^{++} release resulting in PSE meat
- Combination of high temperature and low ultimate pH at post-mortem causes denaturation of specific sarcoplasmic proteins of the affected pig muscles especially enzyme creatine phosphokinase (CP)
- Practically, lack of CP cause accumulation of ADP and inorganic phosphate in the muscle causing speeding up the post-mortem glycolysis
- Application of electrical stimulation just after the slaughter to the carcasses of large ruminant increased the ATP-ase activity and thus, enhanced rate of pH reduction during post-mortem glycolysis

- Application of pressure also causes release of Ca^{++} ions from the SR and stimulate myofibrillar ATP-ase which leads to further stimulation of Ca++-activated ATP-ase of the sarcoplasmic reticulum and thus, acceleration of the post-mortem glycolysis
- The role played by the sarcoplasmic proteins in the water-holding capacity (WHC) becomes negligible since these proteins get precipitated irreversibly even at normal ultimate pH
- WHC and pH are directly proportional
- WHC is lowest at the ultimate pH for a particular muscle and it is likely to increase during conditioning (ageing) of meat
- This is due to high osmotic pressure developed as result of disintegration of larger protein molecules (proteolysis) into minute chains

Rigor mortis

- Muscles become unstretchable as the post-mortem glycolysis continues-- muscle stiffening --referred to as rigor mortis
- The commencement of rigor mortis is associated with the exhaustion of muscle ATP-- the disappearance of ATP leads to formation of firm actomyosin complex by the binding of actin and myosin
- Initially, the muscle stiffness indicating formation of rigid actomyosin commences at low speed (the delay period) followed by high speed (the fast phase) and finally, extensibility persist at a low level

Development of formation of actomyosin progresses:

i. Slowly at the start– known as the 'Delay Period'
ii. Thereafter, with high speed- known as the 'Fast Phase'
iii. Little extensibility persist at a fixed level

- The commencement of the fast phase of rigor mortis at a particular temperature is dependent on the availability of ATP which is gradually utilized by the active non-contractile ATP-ase activity of myosin
- Initially, ATP level is replenished for short time after the slaughter of the animal by the combination of the ADP and creatine phosphate (CP)
- However, once the CP is exhausted, the ATP level goes down effectively
- This situation will arise earlier if the glycogen reserve is low however even if the glycogen level is ample, the ATP generation through the glycolysis cannot maintain ATP to a level enough to inhibit the formation of actomyosin
- If immediately prior to slaughter, the animal experiences struggling, it will decrease its glycogen content leading to faster arrival of the fast

phase of rigor-mortis and similar situation happens in the cases of starvation, insulin tetany

- The arrival of rigor mortis is characterized by reduced WHC
- The drop in WHC is not only contributed by the low ultimate pH (that is also the isoelectric point of the muscle proteins) and denaturation of the sarcoplasmic proteins
- It is important to emphasize that this is not due solely to the drop in pH (and the consequent approach of the muscle proteins to their iso-electric point) or to denaturation of the sarcoplasmic proteins but low WHC is also due to the formation of actomyosin in the absence of ATP

Water is present in muscles in two phases or environments

I. **'Bound' water (lesser quantity of water)**

II. **'Free' water (greater quantity of water is 'free')**

- The quantity of 'bound' water remains same during the arrival of rigor mortis
- However, the 'free' water moves constantly to the other environment initiated by the cross-bonding of actin and myosin (actomyosin formation)
- After the completion of rigor mortis, the muscle will remains hard and unstretchable if there is no contamination with microorganism and hence, the 'resolution' of rigor will not take place
- On the other hand, phenomena of muscle shortening during rigor mortis occurs only due to involvement of small number of the muscle fibres and this muscle shortening is permanent and can be differentiated from physiological contraction
- 'Rigor shortening' intensifies at more than 20 °C temperature whereas 'cold-shortening' is distinctly noticeable at less than 10–15 °C temperatures if the muscle pH is more than 6.2

Types of on-set of rigor mortis

I. **Acid rigor:** is observed in restrained animals having a lengthy delay period and a smaller fast phase and in stressed animals having a very short delay period. At body temperature, muscle inextensibility is associated with muscle shortening

II. **Alkaline rigor:** is observed in animals having quick onset of muscle stiffening and at room temperature, it is characterized by muscle shortening

III. Intermediate type: is observed in starved animals having very short delay period but the rapid phase is not short and little muscle shortening is noticed

- The former (rigor shortening) is noticed immediately prior to onset of full inextensibility in rigor mortis whereas the cold shortening is observed comparatively earlier
- Normally, ATP is essentially needed by the sarcoplasmic reticulum to propel Ca^{++} ions from the sarcoplasm but the reduction in ATP generation during the commencement of rigor mortis causes escape of Ca^{++} ions again towards the sarcoplasm and thus, the contraction mechanism is activated
- This phenomena describes the partial shortening taking place during 'normal' rigor and the great contraction occurring during 'cold-shortening' in which the capability of the sarcoplasmic reticulum pump to recover the Ca^{++} ions is highly reduced due to low temperature
- The myosin S-1 heads interacts with the actin filaments and enhances its inclination (through troponin C) for Ca^{++} ions as the ATP level reduces significantly during post-mortem at the S-1 heads and thus, the sarcomere length reduces at much lower level of Ca^{++} ion compared to *in-vivo*
- The energy required for activation of calpain I autolysis is more compared to its proteolytic action and hence, intensity of tenderization is low at elevated temperature
- Administration of calcium chloride *in-vitro* leads to disintegration of nebulin and the discharge of paratropomyosin (from the A-I junction zone) which combines with actin filaments
- This non-enzymatic action causes breakdown of actin filament and sarcomeres lengthening
- During the post-mortem period, Ca^{++} ions are released from the sarcoplasmic reticulum and thereby, its level increases considerably, bringing meat tenderization during ageing
- Activation of the calpains by higher level of Ca^{++} ions is the chief factor for greater tenderness of meat
- The properties of rigor mortis depends on:
    - Initial quantities of ATP and CP and at the start of rigor-mortis
    - Initial, at the start and ultimate pH
    - Initial and ultimate glycogen reserve
    - ATP-ases and sarcoplasmic reticulum pump activities

- All of the above listed parameters will differ depending on species and type of muscle (intrinsic factors,) environmental temperature and amount of struggling (extrinsic factors)

Unusual rigor mortis: Thaw Rigor

- If the muscle undergoes freezing rapidly while the level of muscle ATP is still high (at the pre-rigor level), such meat upon thawing suffers from an extremely rapid ATP breakdown rate and speedy commencement of rigor mortis ('thaw rigor')
- Muscle undergoing thaw rigor might shrink to 50% of its original length and fluid/liquid is exudated from the muscle known as drip loss
- On freezing and thawing, the contractile actomyosin ATPase is stimulated
- This shows the failure of the sarcoplasmic reticulum pump to retake calcium ions efficiently in these situations
- There are other reasons for thaw rigor apart from the chemical reactions resulting in the formation of actomyosin and resultant muscle contraction in rigor mortis
- The most pertinent reason is in the pattern of nucleotides
- Once ATP is split into inorganic phosphate (Pi) and ADP, the ADP undergoes dephosphorylation and deamination to generate inosine monophosphate (IMP) and further, IMP becomes dephosphorylated to generate inosine
- After that, ribose is broken down from inosine generating hypoxanthine
- However, little amount of ADP undergoes only deamination, synthesizing inosine diphosphate and nucleotides are resynthesized with the aid of enzymes found in muscle for example IMP undergoes condensation with aspartic acid to form adenylsuccinic acid
- Release of ammonia indicates onset of muscle contraction (stiffening) in rigor mortis
- The pre-rigor - characterized by low level of ADP and fairly high level of ATP
- Post-rigor - characterized by high level of IMP and very small quantity of inosine, hypoxanthine, ADP, ATP, IDP and ITP

[illegible]

[illegible] (ageing (tenderisation)). [illegible]

[illegible] at Thaw Rigor

- [illegible]
- [illegible]
- [illegible]

- The process [illegible] characterized by low level of [illegible] and fairly rapid loss of ATP.
- [illegible] characterized by high level of [illegible] MP and [illegible] small quantity [illegible] ATP.

13

Conditioning and Tenderization of Meat

Introduction

Storage of fresh meat without microbiological degeneration at temperature more than freezing point of meat is known as 'conditioning' or 'ageing' and it is said to enhance tenderness and flavor of the meat

Conditioning is also known as ageing or proteolysis of meat

- In the initial 24–36 h after the slaughter, glycolysis is the prevailing reaction going on during post-mortem
- The organization of the contractile proteins can only be conserved by the constant supply of ATP (energy source)
- But ATP supply becomes scarce with the passage of time after death and denaturation of the proteins starts
- Denaturation is a physical or intramolecular reorganization without involving hydrolysis of the bonds occurring between the various amino acids of the polypeptide proteins chains
- Denaturation is characterized by heightened reactivity of different chemical groups, a modification in molecules shape or size, reduced solubility and lost biological reactivity in cases of enzymes or hormones
- In the course of post-mortem conditioning, proteins are prone for denaturation due to lower pH than *in-vivo*, temperatures more than 25 °C or less than 0 °C, dehydration and higher non-physiological salt levels
- Connective tissue proteins such as collagen and elastin do not undergo denaturation during conditioning
- This is indicated by the failure to detect soluble, hydroxyproline-bearing molecules pointing towards non-proteolysis of collagen and elastin
- If collagen is denatured by heating at 60–70 °C for 20–25 min, hydroxyproline-bearing molecules are liberated due to constant non-enzymatic degradation
- Usually, proteolysis occurs only after the protein denaturation

- Myofibrillar and sarcoplasmic proteins experience denaturation of different levels in the course of post-mortem conditioning
- If the meat is cooked just after slaughter and before the commencement of rigor mortis, muscles will be soft and tender
- During this period, the major proteins such as actin and myosin of the myofibril are separated and myosin could be extracted using higher ionic strength
- But if the meat is cooked after the commencement of rigor mortis, the meat becomes tough
- With the progression of the conditioning, the muscles show pliability again (becomes gradually tender on cooking), however, the return of meat pliability is not caused by the severance of actomyosin; inextensibility of muscle remains
- During rigor mortis, actin and myosin are associated with various degrees but this association gets altered in the course of conditioning
- However, there are no proof to show that degradation of actomyosin complex resulted in progression in meat tenderness
- If stress is applied on post-rigor muscles, its lengths are increased
- Lengthening of muscles is dependent on the modifications in the extracellular components such as in the sarcolemma or collagen or mucopolysaccharide of the ground substance and these changes starts with the onset of rigor mortis
- The ability to extract total myofibrillar proteins at high ionic strength reduces by nearly 75% with the commencement of rigor mortis
- However, during conditioning at 2 °C, the extractability increases again to a level that could surpass the starting value
- It is important to note that apart from prevalence of actomyosin, α-actinin, tropomyosin, and the troponin are also included in the extractable myofibrillar proteins at high ionic strength
- Conditioning causes detachment of actin filaments from the Z-line with which actin is joined with the help of tropomyosin and zeugmatin and this association is more fragile than with myosin
- In the course of conditioning/ageing, the Z-lines present in 'white' muscles are more prone to break down compared to those in the 'red' muscles
- Therefore, Z-lines are modified more quickly in rabbit and pork muscles compared to in the large ruminants and higher in semitendinosus than in psoas muscles

- It is important to note that the bovine semitendinosus muscle has nearly triple the activity of CASF (calpains) as in psoas muscle
- It is also worth to note that 'white' muscles are much less vulnerable to 'cold shortening' than 'red' muscles and this is due to higher capability of 'white muscles to regulate intramuscular concentrations of Ca^{++} ions because of a highly efficient sarcotubular system

Effect of ultimate pH on myofibrillar protein during aging

- The ultimate pH of the meat influences the myofibrillar proteins extractability in the way that if the ultimate pH is more, it causes higher extractability
- Similarly, post-mortem temperature affects this significantly: higher temperature causes reduced extractability
- This happens partially because of sarcoplasmic proteins precipitation on the myofibril
- Actomyosin is denatured a little *in-situ* in course of post-mortem glycolysis
- The amount of myofibrillar proteins shortening occurring during the onset of rigor mortis shows the modifications taking place in myofibrillar proteins during the post-mortem which is also indicated by myofibrillar proteins extractability and its tenderness
- If rigor mortis of muscle extends for longer period of time, the formation of actomyosin complex will be little owing to cross bonding and overlapping of actin and myosin at lesser places. This type of meat will be tender on cooking
- Contrary to this, if the rigor mortis is of short duration, significant muscle contraction (shortening) will take place owing to strong and rigid actomyosin complex formation between the actin and the myosin filaments
- Cross bonding will occur at several point and meat will become fairly tough on cooking
- Usually, instead of two extremes that are discussed above, muscle experiences intermediate type of rigor mortis in which the overlapping between the actin and myosin, the cross bond formation and the meat toughness are moderate
- It is observed that the muscle which have experienced severe shortening (contraction) at the commencement of rigor mortis, will show least rate of tenderization in the course of conditioning

- The extent of muscle shortening during rigor mortis depends on the temperature
- Sarcoplasmic protein are greatly prone for muscle post-mortem precipitation
- At room temperature, muscle protein of low ionic strength tends to precipitate and this precipitation is further augmented by increasing the temperature and adding acid and salt

Effects of ultimate pH on sarcoplasmic proteins during meat 'aging'

- As the post- mortem glycolysis advances, there is reduction of pH and it reaches acidic level
- The basic sarcoplasmic proteins glyceraldehyde phosphate dehydrogenase gets denatured and binds with the highly acidic myosin and actin resulting in additional increase in actomyosin formation, thereby, leading to dominance of actomyosin ATP-ase during the course of conditioning
- Sarcoplasmic protein precipitation increases as the temperature increases at all the pH and highest level of precipitation occurs at a pH range of 4.8–5.2 at all the temperatures
- While arriving at the usual ultimate pH (5.5) during post-mortem glycolysis, normally, there is little precipitation of the sarcoplasmic protein
- If the temperature during the post-mortem glycolysis is high, it will cause further precipitation
- Enzyme creatine kinase is one of the highest precipitation prone sarcoplasmic proteins found in the muscles of beef, rabbit and pig
- Sarcoplasmic proteins of pig meat affected with PSE condition undergoes extreme precipitation during post-mortem glycolysis resulting in appearance of pale and exudative meat
- In PSE condition, low pH and high temperature both cause precipitation of sarcoplasmic proteins on to myofibril proteins (actin & myosin) and thereby, reducing their extractability and water holding capacity (WHC)
- Temperature range 37 and 45 °C is considered critical temperature as the high ultimate pH could not retain sarcoplasmic proteins in solution above this temperature range
- PSE affected pigs generally have high body temperature compared to normal just after the slaughter

- Once ultimate pH is reached, apart from changes in the sarcoplasmic proteins, there are other changes in the nature of sarcoplasmic components too
- Myoglobin, a sarcoplasmic protein and chief muscle pigment, gets denatured and enhances the oxidation of iron in it to the ferric form (metmyoglobin) which appears brown
- This is a quite significant change occurring at the cut surface of the meat which is exposed to air
- Desiccation is another factor which can start the denaturation and discoloration, particularly at meat points having comparatively low ultimate pH
- Low ultimate pH is also related with remaining activity in the oxygen utilizing enzymes (succinic dehydrogenase and cytochrome oxidase)
- The most crucial outcome of post-mortem protein denaturation with relation to meat quality is the reduced water-holding capacity (WHC) of meat which is a more widespread property than discoloration
- It is important to note that the lowest WHC of the major meat proteins occurs at pH 5.4–5.5 which is also the isoelectric point of meat
- Normally, rate of formation of lactic acid from the breakdown of glycogen at a specific temperature will result in pH of 5.5 and therefore, little amount of fluid ('weep'or drip) will be lost by meat
- Evidently, the amount of this fluid ('weep') loss will be little if the ultimate pH reached is high
- The WHC is also partially due to the sarcoplasmic proteins but this influence is lost once these proteins are precipitated at usual ultimate pH and cannot be recovered by application of buffer of high ultimate pH to the muscle
- WHC is least at the ultimate pH for any muscle and it increases as the conditioning progresses
- This might be due to enhanced osmotic pressure brought by the degradation of proteins into smaller peptides
- The muscle proteins causes the release of Na and Ca ions into the sarcoplasm and in exchange, absorb the potassium ions after the first 24 h.
- Absorption of more quantity of K^+ ions on the muscular proteins results in increased charge on muscle proteins and hence, WHC increases

Proteolysis

- Denatured proteins are likely to be attacked by proteolytic enzymes
- Conditioning is closely related with the rise in tenderness which is due to enhancement of water-soluble nitrogen as a result of the release of peptides and amino acids from protein molecules
- There is some conflict regarding the proteins which experiences proteolysis during the meat conditioning at temperatures above the freezing point

Proteolysis of connective tissue during aging of meat

- The connective tissue present in skeletal muscle such as the collagen and elastin do not undergo proteolysis during conditioning.
- No increase in water-soluble hydroxyproline-containing molecules is found
- There is no proteolysis of the collagen present in meat during conditioning because such breakdown would require collagenase which would degrade the triple helix structure of collagen at the region of tropocollagen
- However, lysosomal enzymes are present which cleave the cross links present between the triple chains of collagen at the telopeptide region of collagen
- With the progression of meat tenderness, there is simultaneous rise in the concentration of free β- glucuronidase
- β- glucuronidase enzyme can degrade the mucopolysaccharide found in the ground substance or carbohydrate moieties present in collagen
- One of the points of binding of carbohydrate to collagen is the ε-amino group of lysine; and the ε-aminoglycosylamines are perhaps responsible for binding collagen to the ground substance
- In the course of conditioning, proteoglycans present in the basement membrane and the perimysium are broken down
- Hence, it is summarized that degradation of carbohydrate and peptide bonds is responsible of enhanced tenderness in conditioning

Proteolysis of meat proteins by CALPAIN

- The ability of the sarcoplasmic reticulum to store Ca^{++} ions reduces during the course of conditioning
- Clearly, the post-mortem discharge of Ca^{++} ions from the sarcoplasmic reticulum during conditioning brings about the alteration in the

myofibrillar proteins and these changes are operated through water-soluble enzymes

- These enzymes are known by different nomenclatures such as
  - Calcium-activated sarcoplasmic factors (CASF), calcium-activated neutral proteinases (CANP), calcium-dependent proteinases (CDP) or **calpains**
- The calpains are Ca^{2+} dependent proteinases
- 10 of calpain isoenzymes are intensely associated with the tenderization of meat during conditioning/ageing by acting on nebulin and desmin structures
- The calpains are suppressed by the protein called calpastatin
- Calpastatin inhibits calpains due to its helix sequences which prevents calpains binding to membranes
- The calpains breakdown desmin and loosen the connection of α-actinin to the Z-disc
- In the same way, tropomyosin and M-line protein are also disintegrated
- Troponin T undergoes proteolysis during the course of conditioning of beef muscles
- CASF disintegrates the 'gap filaments'
- The calpain proteolysis complex does not affect the actin or myosin because it is confined to the region of Z-line
- During conditioning of *L. dorsi* muscle (at 0 °C for 14 days), simultaneous rise in myofibrillar fragmentation was observed which is used as index of conditioning changes
- During the commencement of reduction of pH, calpains remain inactivated because of its binding to the inhibitor, calpastatin
- However, this prohibitory action decreases as the pH reduction continues and is reduced significantly when pH falls to 5.5 from 6 pH as the calpastatin is proteolyzed by the stimulated calpains
- At first, calpain I action brings the tenderization of meat
- Later on calpain II is activated and causes meat tenderization and it also prevents the self-destruction of calpains by autolysis
- Activation energy required for the calpain I autolysis is more than its proteolysis action and hence, low level of tenderization takes place at higher temperatures

- Calcium chloride introduction *in-vitro* results in nebulin fragmentation and the discharge of paratropomyosin from the A-I junction area which binds to actin proteins
- This non-enzymic action causes disintegration of actin filament and thus, the sarcomeres get lengthened
- During post-mortem, the constant outpouring of Ca^{++} ions from the sarcoplasmic reticulum is responsible for the meat tenderization during conditioning/ageing
- Maximum progression in tenderization is caused by the activation of the calpains by the Ca^{++} ions
- Meat conditioning at 3 to 15 °C causes troponin T proteolysis and rise in meat tenderness
- Though troponin T proteolysis is good indicator of progression of conditioning, other reasons must be taken into account

Lysosomal enzymes (Cathepsins)

- There is another proteolytic enzyme system associated with the meat conditioning called lysosomes
- Contrary to the calcium-activated sarcoplasmic factors (calpains) having optimal pH at more than 6 pH, the cathepsins (B, D, H and L) of the lysosomes have optimal pH at less than 6
- Of these,
    - Cathepsin H is unable to breakdown myofibrillar proteins
    - Cathepsin D is able to disintegrate myofibrillar proteins at lower than 5 pH but its activity at pH 5.5 (ultimate pH) is little during post-mortem ageing
    - Both cathepsins B and L can breakdown these proteins in post-mortem muscle
- Cathepsin L is the most essential lysosomal proteolytic enzyme during conditioning
- It quickly disintegrates troponins T and I, and C and gradually, disintegrates titin (connectin), nebulin, α-actinin, tropomyosin, actin and the light and heavy chains of myosin. Its activity is faster at ultimate pH (pH 5.5)

Meat Tenderness

- Meat tenderness is one of the important meat properties affecting meat acceptability and rebuying intention of the customers

- It is the most essential sensory characteristic of meat for determining customers choice and acceptability
- Knowledge about tenderization process is needed to optimize meat storage and its industrial processing
- Keeping meat at 0 °C to 3 °C causes required alteration in meat fibres brought by the proteolytic enzymes called as "conditioning" or "ripening" or "ageing"
- Tenderized meat-- marked increase in flavour, juiciness and tenderness of the meat.
- Usually, 8 to 11 days storage is considered optimum conditioning period
- Tenderization of meat involves a complicated physicochemical (comprising pH and ionic strength interplay) and biochemical (comprising proteolytic enzymes) processes in which the myofibrillar structure is softened and the cellular integrity is vanished
- During conditioning, proteolytic degradation of cytoskeletal proteins is the main factor responsible for tenderization of meat

Meat proteolytic systems involved in meat tenderization:

1. Lysosomal proteases (cathepsins)
2. Calcium-dependent proteases (calpains), and
3. Proteasomes

- The action of calpains in meat tenderization is well established
- The action of the cathepsins is restricted to initial some days
- The action of proteasomes is conflicting in meat tenderization

Meat tenderization involves two processes

i. Protein Denaturation
ii. Proteolysis

i. Protein Denaturation

- Post-mortem denaturation because of low pH than those in vivo
- Physical or intramolecular rearrangement, loss of biological activity, change in molecular shape and size

ii. Proteolysis

Proteins which are denatured are prone to degradation by the proteolytic enzymes:

A. Calpains
B. Cathepsins
C. Proteosomes

A. By calpain System

During ageing, sarcoplasmic reticulum becomes unable to hold Ca^{++}

↓

Discharge of Ca^{++} ions

↓

Activation of calcium-activated sarcoplasmic factor (CASF): calpains

↓

Degradation of Troponin T (above pH 6), Z-lines (desmin), connectin ("gap filament"), M-line proteins and tropomyosin

CASF (calpains) acts on

i. Troponin T (at more than pH 6)
ii. Z-lines (desmin)
iii. Connectin, "gap filament"
iv. M-line proteins and tropomyosin

- At ultimate pH of 5.5, cathepsins or lysosomal enzymes becomes activated and causes disintegration of actin and myosin filaments

B. By cathepsins system (Lysosomal enzymes)

Lysosomal enzymes (including cathepsins B, D and L) act on

i. Troponins T and I (below pH 6) and C-protein
ii. Myosin (heavy and light chain), actin, tropomyosin, α-actinin, nebulin and titin
iii. Cross-links of non-helical telopeptides of collagen
iv. Mucopoplsaccharides of ground substance

C. Proteasomes

- A third cause of meat proteolysis during condition is proteasomes
- These enzymes are located in a big complex (MW about 700 kDa) consisting of minimum three separate sub-units and each sub-units showing distinct proteolytic action against hydrophobic, basic and acidic amino acid
- Theses enzymes are referred as 'multicatalytic protease complex' or proteasome and its 20S component quickly proteolyse myofibrillar proteins

- Proteasome activity continues during post-mortem and its activity starts after the action of μ and m-calpains is over and takes part in the second phase of proteolysis of denatured proteins
- The proteins of connective tissue and the myofibrils do not undergo appreciable proteolysis during conditioning
- The substantial increase of soluble components of protein degradation during meat conditioning are derived from the sarcoplasmic proteins and not from connective tissue and myofibrillar proteins
- Utmost essential point to be taken into account is that all the above mentioned facts related to meat conditioning is applicable to a usual ultimate pH of nearly 5.5
- The degree of proteolysis lowers as the ultimate pH becomes higher
- The degree of proteolysis is also influenced by temperature, being higher at 37 °C compared to at 5 °C
- This is assumed as there is higher amount of myofibrillar proteins denaturation at the elevated temperature that would resist degradation at low temperature
- Proteolytic action is increased at low ultimate pH by other method
- The lysosomes containing proteolytic enzymes have intact lipoprotein membranes at normal *in-vivo* pH condition
- The lysosomal membrane breaks as the pH reduces during post-mortem, thereby releasing the proteolytic enzymes
- During the course of meat ageing, the myofibrillar structure becomes fragile resulting in transverse fragmentation of sarcomeres
- Weakening of cross-links formed between actin and myosin also adds to enhanced tenderness noticed just after the rigor-mortis period

Flavor development during 'conditioning'/'aging' of meat

- Hypoxanthine and its precursor inosinic acid is responsible for improved meat flavor during conditioning
- As the muscle attains the ultimate pH, ATP is broadly degraded into inosinic acid, inorganic phosphate and ammonia
- Further, depending on time, temperature and pH after the ultimate pH is reached, there is little breakdown of inosinic acid to phosphate, ribose and hypoxanthine
- Optimum organoleptic level is attained during conditioning when the hypoxanthine concentration reaches 1.5–2.0 μmoles/g

- During condition of large ruminants meat, this level is reached after 10–13 days at 0 °C, 4–5 days at 10 °C, 30–40 h at 20 °C and 10–11 h at 30 °C
- The rate of hypoxanthine production is improved by a high ultimate pH
- During conditioning, protein and fat degradation causes liberation of hydrogen sulphide, ammonia, acetaldehyde, acetone and diacetyl which are responsible for flavor development
- Occurrence of fat rancidity greatly affects the meat flavor negatively
- High ultimate pH leads to reduction in oxidative rancidity of fat and myoglobin oxidation
- Besides, the high level of free amino acids derived from proteolysis, the disintegration of numerous peptides contributes to greater concentration of free amino acids
- The dipeptides carnosine and anserine are gradually broken down to β-alanine and histidine during meat conditioning
- For flavor development during ageing, buildup of free amino acids and soluble carbohydrates like glucose (liberated by α-amylase action on glycogen, glucose–6-phosphate (one of the intermediaries in the glycolytic pathway), ribose (from nucleotide degradation)) and other sugars in very small quantities is objectionable
- Reaction between the sugars and protein (Maillard reaction) may take place
- There is little rise in WHC during conditioning but such gain in WHC is offset by the protein denaturation and pH reduction during post-mortem

14

Storage of Fresh Meat

Introduction

- The main objective of food preservation is to avoid food spoilage
- So, the underlying principle behind all the meat preservation technique is providing adverse conditions for the growth and survival of the harmful microbials and such adverse conditions may be provided in the from of heat, cold, high level of salt, increasing acidity or removal of water/ oxygen
- Meat can be preserved by many techniques such as drying, heating, low temperature, curing, addition of chemicals or by application of irradiation and high pressure
- Addition of chemical *i.e.* chemical preservation which is accomplished by smoking is generally done after salting and pickling of meat

Physical changes in stored raw meat

1. Shrinkage
2. Sweating
3. Bloom loss

1. Shrinkage of meat

- Major cause of shrinkage *i.e.* loss in weight is the surface evaporation of water present on meat
- The presence of surface fat, drying of connective tissue and presence of pleura and peritoneum membranes prevent the evaporation
- However, a carcase loses about 1.5–2.0% of its weight by water evaporation during the first 24 h
- Additional loss might happen depending on the relative humidity (RH) in the storage room *i.e.* if RH is low, higher weight loss due to evaporation
- But, maintaining high RH results in moulds growth, therefore precise balance is achieved between the meat storage temperature and RH

- The drying of the membranes present on the meat surface provides the best protection against the spoilage microbes

2. Sweating of meat

- Sweating on meat surface occurs due to lowering of surrounding air temperature by the stored meat preserved at low temperature which is brought outside
- This causes condensation of water vapour on meat surface due to lowering of air temperature less than the dew point

3. Bloom loss of meat

- The colour and appearance of the carcase surface is called bloom
- Bloom is looked through carcase surface consisting of layers of fat, muscle as well as semi-transparent connective tissue membranes
- If meat is exposed to air, muscle pigment assumes brownish colour due to conversion of myohaemoglobin to methaemoglobin (pigment is brown in colour)
- If the carcase surface tissues become wet, it leads to swelling of the collagen present in the connective tissue turning it opaque and thus the meat surface assumes dull and lifeless appearance
- Further, dehydration and oxidation can also result in loss of surface bloom which can be avoided by temperature variations
- Additionally, high RH and free air circulation inside the chilling room ensures durability of meat bloom

Chemical changes in stored meat

- Little breakdown of protein by endogenous enzymes or by the microbes brings about the chemical changes in the meat
- Slowly, the meat odour becomes more prominent but is not objectionable. However, meat may become unpalatable but not disgusting and flavour may be termed as stale
- Nonetheless, chemical changes taking place in fat rather than in muscle is more determining factor for storage life of meat because a little fat rancidity is highly repulsive
- During storage, the meat flavour might be improving due to ageing but simultaneous development of fat rancidity may deteriorate the acceptability of meat and finally make it unacceptable

- Hence, the state of the fat is the major factor controlling the storage life of stored meat

Drying

- The whole process of refrigeration is largely based on the principle of drying, that is, the removal of water available for microbial growth
- Drying is fundamental principle behind refrigeration as it make water unavailable for microorganisms growth
- Similarly, salting withdraws water from meat by osmosis and thereby brings the preservation

Water activity or water availability (a_w)

- Water activity/ water availability (a_w) is the ratio of partial vapour pressure of food items to the partial vapour pressure of the pure water at its surface
- If solutes are added to the food items, water molecules are attracted around these solutes and thus preventing the water availability for microbes
- Microbes except *Staphylococcus aureus* and most moulds are not able to compete with solutes for the water molecules
- Over the usual growth range of microbes, the a_w is little affected by the temperature
- Addition of solutes lowers the a_w (<1) and the highest a_w (1.0) is of pure water
- 0.9% NaCl (w/v) will give 0.99 a_w and 22% NaCl (w/v) will result in reduction of a_w to 0.86
- The a_w may immensely influences the capacity of the microbes under heat
- At 60 °C and a_w of 0.94, the thermal death time (D60) for *Salmonella typhimurium* is 0.18 min
- Microbial growth enhances with increasing a_w and a_w of any microorganism indicates the minimum conditions at which it will grow
- Decreasing the a_w will not definitely destroy the microbes and they will retain the potency to proliferate

Refrigeration

- Combining a high standard of hygiene and packaging with a temperature of −1 to +0.5 °C during storage, transport and display can routinely extend shelf life to 12 weeks

- The preservative action of refrigeration is based on the prevention of multiplication of harmful bacteria, yeasts and moulds by the artificial lowering of the temperature
- The failure of bacteria to grow at or below freezing depends mainly on the removal of the available water as ice; about 70% is removed at -3.5 °C and 94% at -10 °C
- All the microorganisms are not entirely killed either by the blast (slow) or cryogenic (fast) freezing

Meat chilling

- Chilling of meat is mostly done for short duration preservation and meat appearance, flavour and nutritive content is hardly altered by chilling
- Carcases must be chilled instantly after the P.M examination at +7 °C and offals at +3 °C
- Temperature of the meat cutting or deboning room should not exceed +10 °C
- The meat is chilled at around +1 °C in the dark as light encourages fat oxidation leading to free fatty acids release resulting in rancidity development
- The air is maintained in dry condition and relative humidity is kept as low as possible to hinder the formation of moulds
- For initial chilling of warm carcases, temperature is kept below +7 °C and air speed 0.75 m/s
- For meat packed in cartoons, the temperature should be maintained below +3 °C and air speed 0.75 m/s
- For storing offals for more than 72 h, temperature of -10 °C is required

Quick chilling

- *Quick chilling* is decreasing the meat carcase temperature quickly without freezing within 1 h of slaughter
- A relative humidity of about 90%
- *Air circulation rates* 70–110 times the chilling room volume/ h
- For first 24 h, the room temperature should not be less than +5 °C and air circulation rate not more than 1 m/s
- Lower temperature and high air speed--- meat prone for cold shortening
- Pig carcase can tolerate lower temperature and high air speed because carcase size is small and it has skin covering as well as presence of thick subcutaneous fat layer

Advantages of quick chilling

1. It saves time and abattoir space apart from increasing the quantity of carcases to be processed
2. The storage life and quality of meat is improved – bacterial growth is inhibited
3. Shrinkage of meat is reduced
4. The 'bloom' -- enhanced

Cold shortening

- Encountered in quick chilling
- If the meat is chilled (near 10 °C temperature) before it undergoes rigor, pH is above 6.2 and ATP (adenosine triphosphate) is available inside, it would result in severe muscle contraction leading to toughness of meat

Prevention of cold shortening

- Postponing the commencement of chilling—chilling should start 10–12 h post slaughter after passing of rigor when pH would be less than 6.2 and devoid of any muscle ATP
- Chilling not lower than 10 °C in less than 10 h
- Electrical stimulation- its use initiates the rigor quickly

Some specifications for carcase-chilling rooms

- Rails should be at least 0.6 m away from refrigerating unit, room walls and other fixtures of the room
- Header and traffic rails should be 0.9 m from the walls
- The height of the chill rail from floor for beef, pig and sheep/goat carcases should be minimum 3.3, 2.7 and 2 m, respectively.

Vacuum packaging of meat

- Gas-impervious plastic laminate film such as polythene, nylon/ polythene, polyester/ polythene are used to keep primal cuts of meat
- Meat pH should be 5.5-5.8
- Vacuum is created and package is dipped in water bath at 93.5 °C
- The meat packages are stored at between -18 to 1 °C
- Shelf life of up to 2 months

Chilled meat

- Meat suppliers aim to supply the meat with least changes in terms of appearance and palatability of the meat as well as increase in the tenderness of meat
- This is accomplished by keeping the meat chilled without being freezen
- Freezing causes lowering of meat grade
- Hence, meat is chilled at -1.1 °C (just above the meat freezing temperature of – 1.5 °C)
- Shelf life of chilled beef is 35 days – beyond this mould, bacterial slime and taint development
- Storage of chilled meat in CO_2 chambers enhance the shelf life beyond 35 days

Bacterial spoilage of chilled/refrigerated meat

- Mould formation—most common spoilage in chilled meat
- Achromobacter group of bacteria can grow—produces 'cold store taint' or sour
- Small glistening brown droplets on meat surface --- coalesce to form a brownish slime with off odour known as 'cold store taint' or sour
- Number of microbes >30 million/cm^2

Ozonization of chilled/refrigerated meat

- Treatment of meat with ozone at higher concentration inhibits the moulds and yeasts growth
- Addition of ozone to chilling room air destroys surface microorganism and removes stale odour developed in chilling room
- Ozonization is effective to obviate taint produced due to oil and fruit in imported frozen meat
- But ozonization leads to discolouration of lean meat and oxidation of fat

Use of carbon dioxide gas for chilled/refrigerated meat

- Mould growth is inhibited
- Mould growth is completely inhibited at 0 °C if 40% CO_2 concentration is used
- But anaerobes and lactic acid bacteria are almost not affected
- CO_2 inhibits highly aerobic bacteria, yeasts and moulds
- In 10% CO_2 concentration, the shelf life of meat is doubled at 0 °C than in ordinary air

Freezing of meat

- Meat is frozen stored at -18 °C
- The freezing point of meat varies from -1 to -1.5 °C
- During freezing, ice crystal are formed within the muscle from water present inside the muscle
- The ice crystals size and resultant meat quality is determined by the rate of freezing
- Slow freezing causes the formation of large size ice crystals located outside the muscle fibres and these larger size crystals are formed while passing the temperature range between −0.5 to −4 °C and so, this temperature range is called *zone of maximum ice formation*
- When meat is kept at this temperature range, the size of ice crystals becomes large
- These large size ice crystals damage the muscle fibres and the drip loss will be higher on thawing of such meat
- If freezing is done quickly to lower temperature than −4 °C, the ice crystals formed are of smaller size and remain inside the muscle fibres
- If drop in temperature is too fast, ultramicroscopic ice crystals are formed and they are smaller than the size of muscle fibres inside which they are formed
- These smaller ice crystals do not damage the muscle fibres thus drip loss will be minimum upon thawing such meat
- Hence, *quick freezing of meat* is preferred

Changes in frozen meat

Freezing causes two undesirable changes in meat

1. Loss of globulin and albumen proteins (muscle plasm) solubility
   - Freezing at below -2 °C leads to formation of ice crystals resulting in increase in the concentration of these proteins and loss of their solubility
   - Lost solubility is not regained by thawing
2. Formation of ice crystal inside the meat—the size of the ice crystals affects the 'weeping'/'drip' loss on thawing

'Weeping' or 'drip' loss

Thawing of frozen meat results in oozing of blood-stained liquid from the meat, formation of dew on meat surface and watery discharge, all are called 'Weeping' or 'drip' loss. Drip is comprised of water, salts, proteins and damaged blood cells

- Weeping is an adverse phenomenon occurring due to the rupture of the muscle fibres and tissues by large ice crystals and partially by irrevocable alterations in the muscle plasm
- If the size of ice crystals formed is large during freezing, it damages the muscle cells and therefore, 'weeping' or 'drip' shall be more
- Slow freezing- large size ice crystals formation- higher drip loss on thawing
- Fast freezing- small size ice crystals formation- lower drip loss on thawing
- The drip quantity is higher in beef compared to mutton, lamb or pork
- Drip loss is minimal if very slow thawing is done
- Ultimate temperature reached after thawing has the great influence on drip loss
- It is a fact that the loss of drip will be more from the muscles and rigor mortis will set earlier if the ATP present in meat muscle is utilized at rapid rate
- Hence, slowing down the ATP breakdown and resultant delay in rigor mortis will finally lead to lower free fluid to be released as drip fluid on future freezing and subsequent thawing

Storage life of frozen meat

- Freezing turns the meat dry, rancid and lowers its taste
- Most significant change—development of rancidity by degrading fat releasing glycerine and free fatty acids
- Beef can be frozen stored for one year under proper condition
- Beef has the longest storage life and pork has the shortest (6 months); lamb 8-9 months; mutton 8-9 months

Freezing by liquid nitrogen

Freezing meat using liquid nitrogen called *cryogenic freezing* results in less drying of meat and texture, flavour, aroma and nutritive content of the meat is improved compared to traditional freezing using cold air

Freeze-drying or lyophilisation of meat

- This is used to remove water from the meat
- Firstly, the meat is sliced or minced (comminuted form) and then frozen
- Meat is kept in freeze dryer where vacuum is created causing water to evaporate even when the temperature is low

- Once drying is over, meat is packed in complete water impervious packaging material as the dried meat is highly hygroscopic

Affections of imported meat

1. Brine staining
2. Freezer burn

1. Brine staining

- Meat stored in refrigeration rooms having imperfect joints or leakage in brine circulation system might get covered with calcium chloride solution
- This covering produces dull or pale greenish colour on the carcase surfaces- '**Brine staining**'
- The stain penetrates deep and darkens the muscular tissue --- extremely bitter taste
- Trimming of the affect meat part will make it fit for consumption
- Sea water contamination—only salty taste, no bitterness, and no pale green colouration

2. Freezer burn

- This is observed on the external surface of frozen offals, particularly the liver, hearts and kidneys and is due to the superficial tissue dehydration
- Occasionally, it is encountered on uncovered stored carcase surface kept near the opening of cooling dust
- Dehydration or crystallization on the offals surface—soft and spongy with yellowish withered patches—wastage due to drip loss (3-7%)
- Offals become insipid and unpalatable on cooking--- so condemnation
- This defect can be avoided by suitable wrapping or cryogenic freezing to -24 °C

Effect of freezing on pathogenic micro-organisms and parasites

- Only few bacteria are killed by freezing
- Freezing temperature arrest the bacterial growth and proliferation
- Freezing cannot render infected carcase harmless for human ingestion
- Slow or fast freezing do no destroy the bacteria
- Anthrax bacilli and *Salmonella* can withstand -130 and -175 °C, respectively for 3 days
- Tuberculosis bacteria can remains active in -10 °C frozen carcase even after two years

- Swine fever virus remains infective for 73 days and viable for 1500 days in chilled/frozen carcase
- FMD virus remains viable for 76 days in chilled/frozen carcase
- Freezing has valuable effect on some parasitic infections
- Pork meat containing *cysticercus cellulosae* could be rendered safe for human consumption if kept for 4 days at -10.5 to - 8 °C
- Beef containing *cysticercus bovis* if stored at not higher than - 6.5 °C for 3 weeks or at temperature not surpassing -10.5 °C for 2 weeks could become safe for consumption
- Keeping the infected pig carcase at 15 °C for 20 days or use of quick freezing for 24 h at -18 °C kills the *Trichinella* cysts

Vacuum packing

- Primal cuts or meat cuts having pH 5.5–5.8 are kept in gas impervious plastic film laminates such as polythene, nylon/ polythene, polyester/ polythene at 2–4 °C and vacuum packed
- The packages are stored at temperature range of -18 to 1°C
- Meat muscle respiration utilizes the left over oxygen and thus, CO_2 level rises
- Lack of water and air significantly prohibits the microbial growth
- However, due to absence of air, myoglobin turns bluish although it retains back the red colour when the pack is opened as the oxygen converts the myoglobin to oxymyoglobin
- Meat with high quality in terms of bacterial count could have shelf life of up to 3 months

Basic systems of vacuum packing: Two

1. 'Cryovac' system: air inside the meat packs is drawn out by vacuum and then the packs are carried through hot water dip or tunnel having hot air

   The advantage of this packing:

   i. Drip fluid is reduced

   ii. Risk of tearing of the packages are reduced
2. Air is removed by vacuum followed by no heat shrinkage

Modified atmosphere packaging (MAP) of meat

- In MAP, meat is kept in highly impervious packaging material followed by sucking out air using vacuum, filling the packages with mixture of desirable gases and finally sealing it

- Gases are selected so as to hinder the microbial multiplication and increases the shelf life of meat
- 10–50% carbon dioxide is added which inhibits the growth of many micro-organisms that cause spoilage of refrigerated meats
- Proliferation of many harmful microorganism in chilled meat is prevented by filling 10–50% carbon dioxide gas in the meat packages
- Further, filling of 20–50% oxygen in the meat packages ensures cherry red colour of myoglobin due to oxygenation
- Packaging material for MAP must be gas–impermeable to maintain the desired air composition
- High level of CO_2 prevents moulds proliferation
- However, CO_2 is not able to prevent facultative bacterial growth and lactic acid bacteria and anaerobes practically remains undisturbed
- Contrarily, CO_2 prevents the growth of highly aerobic microbes, yeasts and moulds
- 40% concentration of CO_2 gas at 0 °C entirely inhibits the mould development

15

Physicochemical Parameters of Meat

Physicochemical parameters of meat

1. Moisture, ash and fat content

- Meat samples are dried at 105 °C for 24 h for determining the moisture content and for ash content analysis, samples are burned at 525 °C
- Fat determination is done by acidic hydrolysis of the sample
- Sample is boiled initially and then cooled and later, it is filtered, washed and dried
- Thereafter, petroleum ether is used to extract the fat
- Ether is evaporated and the remnant is dried and weighed

2. Protein content

- Often, protein in meat sample is estimated using Kjeldahl method
- The protein content is determined by multiplying the nitrogen content in the meat sample by an appropriate conversion factor
- Strong acid is used to digest the meat sample and the released nitrogen is measured by proper titration technique
- Then, the protein quantity of the sample is determined from the nitrogen concentration of the meat
- Kjeldahl method does not determine the protein content in straightway manner; a conversion factor (F) is required to convert the nitrogen content to protein content
- Usually, a conversion factor of 6.25 (corresponding to 0.16 g nitrogen/g of protein) is used for several food samples

3. Meat colour

- Colour is one of the most significant factors affecting the consumers' judgement regarding meat purchase
- Colour analysis can be performed using a colorimeter calibrated for internal light D56 against a reference

- The meat samples are evaluated for L* (lightness), a* (redness/greenness) and b* (yellowness/blueness) values
- The colour space is organized in a cube form. The L* axis runs from top to bottom in a straight line
- The L* value for any sample can range from 0 to 100
- The maximum value for L* that can be recorded for a sample is 100 which indicates a perfect reflecting surface (white surface) signifying the complete white colour of the meat sample
- And the minimum value that can be obtained for L* is 0 which shows that the meat sample is complete black
- The a* and b* axes have no fixed value range and a* and b* values may be a positive or negative number
- If the value of a* obtained for a meat sample is positive number, it shows redness of the meat sample
- Higher the positive a* value of any meat sample, more red it will be in appearance
- If the value of a* obtained for a meat sample is negative number, it shows greenness of the meat sample
- Similarly, positive b* value for a sample indicates its yellowness while negative b* value indicates the blueness
- Higher positive b* value for any meat sample show that the meat sample is more yellow in appearance
- There are delta values related with this colour scale
- ΔL*, Δa*, and Δb* show differences between standard and sample in L*, a*, and b* values

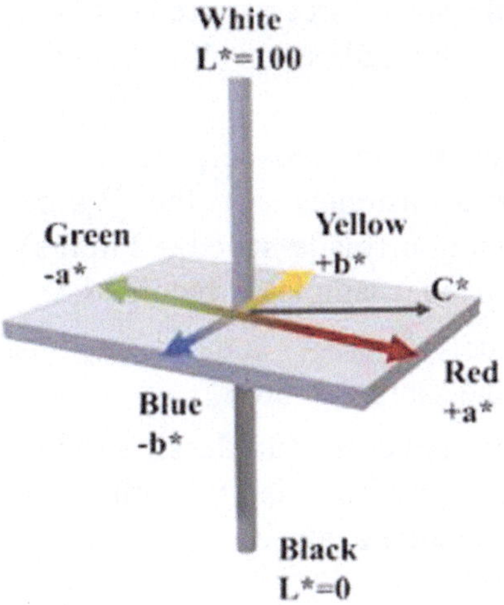

Fig. 1. Colour coordinates of Hunter Lab colour system L*, a*, and b* (*Source*: Jin, Y., Xu, J., Li, Y., Zhao, Z., Chen, M., Lu, L., & Li, L. (2022). Rheological properties, shape stability and compressive strength of 3D printed colored cement composites modified by needle-like pigment. *Additive Manufacturing*, *57*, 102965)

4. pH

- The pH of the meat samples are recorded with the help of digital pH meter
- Approximately 5 g of meat sample is added to 45 ml of distilled water and the mixture is homogenized using laboratory blender and the pH is noted down
- The pH value of meat affects the shelf life, tenderness, colour and WHC and provides valuable information about exposure of animals to preslaughter stress
- Low ultimate pH promotes denaturation of myoglobin, sarcoplasmic and myofibrillar proteins and thus accelerates the loss of their extractability
- More protein is extracted at higher pH
- Generally, if the pH of the meat is high, its WHC capacity is more

5. Texture analyses

- The firmness, elasticity as well as breaking point of meat products can be obtained through a texture analyser
- For the firmness and elasticity measurements, a 36-mm cylindrical stainless steel probe is used whereas for breaking force, tensile grips with a capacity 35 mm is used to hold the specimens, which consisted of slices of meat (40×40×1mm size)

- For determining the shear force required to cut the meat samples, sample piece parallel to the fibre direction (1.4 cm in diameter) are incised from the meat sample
- The meat samples are sheared perpendicular to fibre direction using texture analyzer accustomed for the Warner-Bratzler shear force (WBSF) determination (blade speed = 2 mm/s). The average of shear force (*N*) from the meat samples is recorded
- Texture profile analysis (TPA) is determined using compression probe by compressing the sample to 60%
- Hardness (kg), cohesiveness (unitless), springiness (mm), gumminess (kg) and chewiness are recorded with the help of computer software attached with the texture analyser

6. Meat tenderness

- Although a part of the texture profile, meat tenderness is closely related with ultimate pH (pH_u) of meat
- Aging of meat having high ($pH \geq 6.2$) and low ($pH \leq 5.79$) pH_u are found to be suitably tender
- Besides, the rate of meat tenderisation is also related with ultimate pH, for example, meat with high pH_u tenderizes more quickly compared to low pH_u meat
- Biochemical changes occurring in muscles during post-mortem are pH dependent
- Several alterations occurring at low and high pH_u meat during post-mortem causes meat tenderisation at both pH_u
- Meat tenderness is resulted due to disruption of the greatly ordered myofibrillar structure caused by proteolysis of major meat proteins after the slaughter of the animal
- Calpains as well as cathepsins enzyme systems are involved in post-mortem proteolysis
- The stoppage of ionic pumps during post-mortem as the ATP supply becomes insufficient leads to building up of sarcoplasmic Ca^{2+} ions to a concentration level that activates μ- and m-isoforms of calpain resulting in myofibrillar proteins hydrolysis
- Additionally, the reduction of muscle pH during post-mortem ageing causes lysosomal membrane to become weak and ultimately, leads to discharge of cathepsins from the lysosomes which in turn hydrolyse the myofibrillar proteins

- Quicker and more extensive degradation and its higher rate are observed in desmin, troponin T, filamin, nebulin and titin in tender meat than in tough meat
- A relationship exists between the meat tenderness and its pH; as the pH_u rises from 5.5 to 6.0, it results in lowering of meat tenderness; this effect then reverses as the pH further rises above 6.0 meaning tenderness increases as the pH_u increases above 6.0

7. Water-holding capacity (WHC) of meat

- WHC is an index of the bound water and is generally measured by estimating the 'loosely held' water which can be removed by pressure or centrifuge, *etc.*
- The ability of meat (myofibril protein) to retain its water or added water when undergoes cutting, grinding or pressing is called WHC
  - WHC influences:
    - Color
    - Texture and firmness of meat
    - Meat palatability
    - Juiciness and tenderness of meat
  - Meat with high WHC will show stronger structure and a dry texture
  - On the contrary, if WHC is low, meat appears soft, moist texture, watery and absence of toughness of meat
  - The most commonly used procedure to determine WHC of a meat sample is the filter-paper press technique

Water-holding capacity (WHC) is measured by

i. Purge/thaw loss
ii. Drip loss and
iii. Cooking loss

i. Purge/thaw loss

Purge (or thawing) loss is recorded by measuring percentage weight differences between initial weight before the commencement of aging and/or freezing and weight of the meat sample at the end

ii. Drip loss

- For assessing drip loss, 40 g of sample is taken in a cube shape
- Sample is kept inside onion net and suspended inside an airtight container for 48 h

- Thereafter, the sample is dried using blotting paper and weighed again
- The difference in initial and final weight is expressed in percentage water loss

iii. Cooking loss

- Cooking loss is measured using the meat sample (2.4 cm thick)
- The meat sample is cooked till internal temperature of 71 °C is attained
- Finally, the weight difference between the initial and final weight of the sample is calculated as percentage cooking loss

The bulk of water in muscle is held either within the myofibrils, between the myofibrils and between the myofibrils and the cell membrane (sarcolemma), between muscle cells and between muscle bundles (groups of muscle cells).

The water present in meat can be divided into three portions:

i. Bound water
ii. Immobilized/entrapped water
iii. Free water

i. Bound water

- Water is a dipolar molecule and is attracted towards the charged entity such as proteins
- The water in muscle cells which is tightly bound to muscle proteins are referred as 'bound water'
- 'Bound water' due to its attachment to muscle protein show very little movement meaning they do not migrate normally to other compartments
- This water resist freezing to a great extent
- The amount of bound water do not varies and if this happens, it happens in post-rigor meat only

ii. Immobilized/entrapped water

- Another part of water that is present in muscles is called as 'entrapped' or 'immobilized' water
- Such water is attached either by steric (space) effect and/or by attraction to the 'bound' water
- This water is contained inside muscle structure and is not bound to muscle protein
- During the initial period of post-mortem, this water cannot move freely from the muscles but it can be removed by drying and it can be frozen

- 'Entrapped'/ 'immobilized' water is greatly influenced by the rigor-mortis and the transformation of muscle to meat
- If muscle cell structure is altered or pH is lowered, this water oozes out as purge

iii. Free water

- 'Free' water is water which can easily move out of muscle
- This portion of muscle water is primarily bound to muscle by weak surface forces
- During the conversion of muscle into meat, the amount of 'entrapped'/ 'immobilized' water is mainly changed
- Keeping large portion of free water within the meat product is the aim of the meat processors

Physico-biochemical factors affecting water holding capacity (WHC)

i. Net charge effect

- The accumulation of lactic acid inside the muscle due to anaerobic glycolysis at the post-mortem stage leads to pH of meat to fall
- As the meat pH attains the isoelectric point (pI) of the myosin protein (pI = *5.4),* the overall charge of the meat protein becomes zero
- This indicates that the numbers of positive and negative charges on the meat protein has become equal
- These positive and negative charges on the muscle proteins attract one another resulting in drop in attraction and holding of water by the proteins and thereby, decline in the quantity of muscle water

ii. Genetic factor

- Rapid pH fall and low ultimate pH results in decline in WHC and resultant excessive purge/drip loss
- Accelerated pH fall leading to ultimate or close to ultimate pH while the carcass is still hot causes muscle protein denaturation and consequently, loss in ability to hold water and thereby, decline in WHC of muscle proteins
- Hence, unacceptably high purge or drip loss is noticed in condition of pale, soft, and exudative meat (PSE meat) which is caused by heritable mutation in the ryanodine receptor/calcium release channel (halothane gene) in the sarcoplasmic reticulum

iii. Steric (space) effect

- Majority of the water found in living muscle cells is present inside the myofibril
- Almost 85% of the water in a muscle cell is contained in the myofibrils
- Majority of this water is held between the spaces arising out of arrangement of the thick and thin filaments inside the myofibril due to capillary forces
- In living muscle, during contraction and relaxation of muscle, sarcomeres length do not change meaning it shows isovolumetric property
- This signifies that the quantity of water held inside the fine structures of myofibrils in the living muscle do not change due to contraction and relaxation of muscle
- But the site of this water may vary due to alteration in the muscle volume during rigor mortis
- With the onset of rigor mortis, actomyosin cross cross-bridges formed between actin and myosin significantly reduces the space available for water to be held by capillary forces

16

Cleaning, Sanitation, Hygiene and Waste Management of Slaughterhouse Plants

Introduction

- The source of contamination of meat plant is largely from the animals entering in the plant
- Severely contaminated hide/skin are the major source of abattoir contamination
- If proper hygiene of employees, equipments and clothing is not followed, then even after skinning 10,000 to 100,000 bacteria/ in^2 can be detected
- Blades of knives can carry 80,000 to 40 millions bacterial per blade & hands of meat operative can have $3x10^9$ bacteria/g of scrapings
- The chance of contamination of carcase is greater at the point of incision and minimum at the farthest point from the incision place

'Scotoma effect' or 'factory-blindness'

- Persons working in any factory or abattoir on routine basis slowly and slowly becomes unaware (mentally 'blind') about any sub-standard hygiene or cleanliness problem existing in the surrounding
- This effect is known as 'scotoma' or 'factory-blindness'
- Effect can be powerful and the any visitors to that factory or abattoir will instantly notice that sub-standard hygiene or cleanliness problem neglected by the persons working there
- The 'scotoma' effect is checked by continuous alertness, training, regular monitoring and examination and internal audition
- Trained persons from outside agency or external auditors can also be brought on regular basis to overcome this effect

Cleaning

Sterilization

- Any physical or chemical process which destroys all the living microorganisms (absence of all life forms)

Disinfectants

- Chemical agents which destroy microorganisms but not essentially its spores

Antiseptic

- Is a substance which deters the proliferation of microbes either by killing it or arresting its activity

Germicide

- Is a substance which destroys the vegetative microbial cells but not necessarily its spores and thus it is similar to disinfectant

Sanitizer

Is a chemical agent which decreases the number of surface contamination with bacteria coming in contact with foods to acceptable bacteriological standards

The chemistry of cleaning

Basically, cleaning is a physicochemical process involving many reactions depending on the following factors:

1. The soil
2. The substrate: Materials of construction
3. Energies of cleaning
4. Chemical and physical reactions of cleaning

1. The soil

- 'Soils' or other dirty deposits gain entry into the premises from the entering animals and other related activities
- Usually, various soil types are found in the same slaughterhouse mixed with other deposits
- Actually, combining with other deposits turns them more tougher, harder, adhering more firmly and finally, more problematic in taking it out from the deposited surfaces
- Important to identify the soils present in each plant area by their origins and by their appearance- important to design the correct cleaning regime

- It is essential to diagnose the type of soil present by its occurrence and appearance in the abattoir- significant since it will help in designing a proper cleaning plan

These product-derived soils include the following:

Fats, oils and greases

- These are triglycerides of fatty acids and can range from waxy solids to liquids
- They are water insoluble and can differ in their structure and characteristics based on:
  - Their origin
  - Various body parts of the same animal species
  - Difference in the animals age and
  - Variations in species
- Fats obtained during dressing of poultry are too waxy and tough to remove than beef tallow
- If exposed to air, fats, oils and greases can modify and get oxidized or polymerized to turn into harder and more tenaciously adhered to the surface
- High temperature results in fats to carbonise and get adhered to stainless steel surfaces
- Fully polymerised oils can turn into nearly plastic in feel and hardness

Proteins

- Are big and complicated molecules and are generally too large that it does not get dissolved easily in water
- Protein possess a particular configuration which gets distorted (denaturation) when undergoes high temperature which makes it more tougher and insoluble
- Aged protein deposits are quite hard

Carbohydrates and starches

- These are also big molecules
- They are insoluble in water, particularly after experiencing heat
- Generally, obtained from plant-derived materials
- Found in different consistencies ranging from soft and powdery to quite hard

Miscellaneous deposits

These deposits include the soils not generated from the core slaughterhouse processes rather they are generated from supply water, any type of corrosion, vehicles and other external things. These deposits are:

- Lime scale formation through water drippings and leakages
- Rust deposits of steel, zinc, aluminium, brass, *etc.*
- Rubber marks from forklift trucks
- Glues from the labels
- Inks and dyes from stamps
- Algal growth in high moisture areas
- Fungus growth in cold moist areas such as close to chiller and freezer and in silicon sealants throughout the abattoir

2. The substrate: Materials of construction

- Stainless steel-- high grade is the excellent selection for several contact surfaces
- Mild steel-- rusting is a problem in humid and salty situations and usually, 0should not be used in abattoirs
- Zinc & aluminium —they are used as protective coating on steel and are questionable due to their vulnerability to strong acids, alkalis, and some fluids
- Terrazzo and concrete--- both are liable to turn out to be porous and cracked if neglected and are prone to corrosion by acids
- Paints and other coatings—differ in their ability to resist chemical attacks and hot or pressurised water: becomes a problem when flaking due to risk of food contamination
  - Chemical-resistant resins can be applied
- Plastics and rubbers too differ extensively
  - These can swell on contact with some detergents, which may affect unhindered running of machinery

3. Energies of cleaning

Fundamentally, there are combination of four factors in cleaning process that affect the cleaning process:

Thermal energy

- It may be hot water or steam
- A rise of 10 °C temperature of a detergent solution, doubles the rate of the chemical reactions of cleaning

Mechanical energy

- Examples of mechanical energy are use of brushes, water jets, turbulent flow in pipes, micro-agitation caused by the bursting of foam bubbles
- In CIP (cleaning- in-place) system, a flow rate of almost 2 m/s is required to cause turbulent flow and prevent laminar flow— results in better cleaning

Chemical energy

- This is determined by the detergent type and its concentration employed

Time

- Time of application of cleaning system ranges from hours in soak cleaning to seconds in tray or crate cleaning

4. Chemical and physical reactions of cleaning

Detergency comprises of physical and chemical reactions which are determined by the soils types to be cleaned and the detergent types applied to cleanse them

Physical reactions

The primary physical reactions are the following:

Wetting

- The first important phase in the removal of the soil
- Displacement of one fluid from a surface by another fluid is termed as wetting
- The displaced fluid might be air or other liquid or semi-liquid such as fat/grease
- The water or a detergent solution might act as displacing fluid
- But water alone lacks wettability to displace several soils types
- Inability to wet a surface results in improper cleaning
- To attain the ability to wet, 'surfactants' or 'wetting agents' are used in combination
- These are organic molecules having different ends
- One end is basically a hydrocarbon known as 'hydrophobic' end
- Whereas, the other end is either ionised to provide a positive or negative charge or made up of oxygen-containing groups--'hydrophilic'end
- The leads to dual-nature molecule accumulating at the interface between the water and the surface and thus, allows wetting

Penetration

- Wetting agents permits the detergents to dislodge air from surfaces and thus allow for deeper penetration of detergents much quicker into the dry deposits than water on its own
- Once the detergent comes into the contact of dry deposits, its active constituents react with soil and dislodge it

Emulsification

- Emulsions are solution of one fluid holding the suspended droplets of another fluid
- By nature, fats, oils and greases will not dissolve in water
- Foremost, the oil requires to be set free from the surface it is holding on
- Wetting is the initial phase in releasing the oil from the surface holding it as detergent weakens the oil–surface attraction and thus, initiates displacement of oil and formation of small droplets
- This whole process hastens if the temperature is more resulting in fat/oil/grease liquefaction and/or high mechanical energy is employed to the soil
- The oil droplets are released from the surface and they float easily
- These droplets have tendency to coalesce and become single bigger drop and to redeposit somewhere else
- To avert the coalescence, surfactants are used which forms a layer on the oil droplets and stabilise the emulsion

Dispersion

- Same as emulsification except that it includes the disintegration and suspension of solid particles instead of fluid droplets
- Often, inorganic compounds like carbonates, silicates, phosphates or special water-soluble charged polymers are employed along with detergent for dispersion which are different than surfactants
- Stable dispersion are formed which are removed by rinsing and do not get settled again
- Stable dispersion are produced by covering the particles with same electric charges which repel each other
- Production of dispersion is mainly important in circulating type of cleaning systems as the slow moving solid particle have tendency to get settled down to form sludge

Solubilisation

- Basically, this process involves turning up of soil constituents into a true solution
- However, by nature, few soil components are water-soluble whereas some others are not and hence require solvents in the detergent solution to make them water-soluble
- These solvents should be stain-free, less toxic and are normally, alcohols, glycols or glycol ethers based
- They aid greatly in dislodging hard, greasy soils which are tough to emulsify
- The solvents go inside the grease and soften or liquefy it

Chemical reactions

The most important chemical reactions are the following:

Proteins and carbohydrates hydrolysis

- These large molecules are built by smaller subunits such as peptides and amino acids are subunits of proteins
- Hydrolysis is the breakdown of larger molecules at the joint of smaller subunits and thus releasing smaller subunits which are water soluble
- Normally, hydrolysis occurs at extreme pH and that is why, acids and alkalis are used in detergents
- Although, hydrolysis involving alkalis are highly effective, deposits of bile proteins found at evisceration area are more susceptible to acid hydrolysis
- In case of old blood stains, alternation of alkaline and acid detergents is very helpful
- For removing old blood stains, alkalis and acid detergents are used alternatively

Fats, oils and greases saponification

- In this type of hydrolysis, when an alkali combines with triglyceride fats, it results in production of water-soluble glycerol and soap
- Practically, the production of soap can be advantageous as it will work as a wetting and emulsification agent or it can be disadvantageous as it causes formation of foam in circulatory cleaning
- Formation of foam is of less problem in hard water but in hard water, scum will be formed with calcium and this will make cleaning less effective

Chelation

- Chelation of insoluble metal ions such as calcium, magnesium and iron
- In the scales already formed on the surface, these ions may be existing and offering spaces for further soil adherence and thus get combined with the deposits itselves
- This chelation may get affected if the water is hard water
- Chelating agents, chelants or sequestrants, combines with theses metal ions in water-soluble cages and thus remove the scale or prevents its formation
- In mixed scale/soil deposits, the disintegration of deposits is highly influenced by chelation
- The classical examples of chelating agents are ethylene diamine tetraacetic acid (EDTA) and gluconate
- Chelants are usually supplemented by substoichiometric chelants which are normally water-soluble charged polymers

Chelants act in two ways

1. They prohibits the formation of microcrystals of scales by obstructing the corners of crystals where scales are formed and thus, compelling the crystals to become circular shape
   - Thus, even if scales are formed, it would be soft and powdery and non-adherent to surfaces
2. They also work as dispersants attaching microcrystals as pearls in a necklace and forcing them from sticking to each other and thus, precipitation is ensured
   - The polymeric chelants do not require to be used in a fixed ratio to the metal ions
   - Their optimal action takes place at lower alkalinity such as during the rinse stage
   - Usually, they do not detach the already formed scales

Oxidation

- Oxidation of coloured materials, starches, *etc.*
- Coloured scales are bleached and some protein or fat scales may be damaged easily
- Normally, chlorine is applied in the form of alkaline sodium hypochlorite

- The chief action of chlorine is as oxidising agent when present in alkaline detergent solution
- In alkaline detergent solution containing chlorine in the form of hypochlorite, both the alkalinity and the chlorine molecules are needed to dislodge scales formed from protein and fat

Corrosion inhibition

- Corrosion takes place when detergents come in contact with aluminium and zinc at extreme pH
- Few chemical constituents can prevent corrosion
- Caustic soda when mixed with silicates does not corrodes aluminium however, there is incremental chance of formation of scales of insoluble calcium silicate

Enzymolysis

- At medium pH, protease, lipase and amylase may be used to make effective special type of detergents
- Enzymes break down the big organic molecules by alkaline or acid hydrolysis
- However, this type of stable detergents are tough to produce

Detergents: its formulation and selection

- Detergents are formulated to eradicate soils
- Sanitizer –a combination of detergent and disinfectant
- Disinfectants are chemicals formulated to kill microorganism but lacks soil removing property
    - Detergent formulation and selection depends on the physical and chemical reactions required from the detergents to dislodge scales
    - If the deposits are highly complex and variable, various different constituents are needed to formulate the detergents
    - Similarly, the detergent formulation depends on the water hardness, temperature and application method, safety of the workers and plant surfaces and its potential effects on effluent system
    - The major constituents of detergents which may/may not be present jointly, are:
        - Alkalis: caustic soda, caustic potash, carbonate, silicate and phosphate

- Acids: phosphoric, nitric, citric, glycolic, sulphamic and hydrochloric
- Chelating agents: EDTA, gluconate, glucoheptonate, citrate and polymers
- Solvents: isopropanol, propylene glycol, butyl diglycol and ethers
- Surfactants: anionic, cationic, non-ionic and amphoteric
- Corrosion inhibitors: organic and inorganic
- Enzymes: protease, lipase and amylase
- Oxidising agents: hypochlorite, isocyanurates and peracids
- Stabilisers
- Viscosity modifiers

Detergents consist of two main categories

I. Soapy detergents

II. Soapless detergents

I. Soapy detergents

Manufactured by heating oil/fat with an alkali (caustic soda)

II. Soapless detergents

- Prepared by sulphonation (reaction with sulphur trioxide) of mineral oils
- Normally in the form of powders or liquids
- Few soapless detergents are manufactured by sulphonating tallow alcohol and by reacting alcohols with ethylene oxide

  - Fats and oils used in making soaps are trigycerides (one molecule of glycerol (gycerine) combined with three molecules of fatty acids)
  - Fats/oils are broken down by caustic soda (NaOH) releasing glycerine and caustic soda combines with fatty acids to form hard soap
  - If potassium is used instead of sodium to react with fats/oils, soft soap are produced as they retain the glycerine in it
  - In water solution, the soap molecules ionizes into two ions; negative charge possessed by carboxylate (hydrophilic) and hence soap is known as anionic surfactant
  - If the electric charge is positive, the surfactant is known as cationic surfactant

- If there are no electric charge, the surfactant is known as non-ionic surfactant
- Enzyme based foam cleaning agents are used to remove protein and fat
- It consists of stabilized enzyme solution and an alkaline builder formulation containing water-conditioning agent
- When enzyme solution and alkaline builder are mixed in equal proportion and diluted (1-2%), it gives a self foaming cleaning solution having emulsifying, penetrating action on fat and disintegrating action on protein due to presence of enzyme
- It expands in volume up to 40 times by incorporating air in it
- While most of the detergents are alkaline, some are acidic based on sulphamic, phosphoric or hydrochloric acids and are used to remove scales (protein and caorbohydrate) formed in the premises

There are four main groups of detergents or surface-active agents

i. Anionic detergents—produce negatively charged ions in solution such as soaps and detergents
ii. Cationic detergents—produce positively charged ions in solution
    - Having good wetting, foaming and emulsifying ability but are weak detergent
iii. Non-ionic detergents--- do not produce any charge insolution
iv. Amphoteric or ampholytic detergents--- depending on the pH of the solution, it produces negative or positive ions in the solution
    - Not used extensively in food industry

Properties of good detergent or cleaning agents are as follows

i. Ability to remove soil from the surfaces
ii. Ability to prevent scale formation in hard water system
iii. Minimum ringing should be required
iv. Maintains relatively stable degrees of acidity or alkalinity
v. Ability to combine with sanitizing agents
vi. Non-toxic
vii. Not tainting to meat and offals
viii. Economical to use
ix. Non-corrosive to surfaces
x. Good biodegradability

Principles of disinfection

- Usually, a decrease of 3–4 logs/cm^2 in total viable count is achieved by cleaning
- For example, if initially, the microbial load was 10^6 CFU/cm^2, it would go down to 10^2–10^3/cm^2 after cleaning
- Hence, disinfectants are used to bring down the microbial load to lower than few hundreds
- Full sterilisation of meat plant surfaces are not required as well as it is not possible

Biocidal active components of disinfectant

- The disinfectants are used to destroy bacteria and other microbials left on the meat contact surfaces after cleaning
- Destruction of microbes are brought about by various methods depending on which constituents are used in the disinfectant

Oxidising disinfectants

- It combines with several organic compound like meat residues and bacteria
- Examples- chlorine, iodophors and peracids
- Quick action and broad spectrum as they destroys living microorganism along with its spores
- Do not have residual action
- Stability is not sure in hot water
- Corrosive on metals and other surfaces
- Low foaming
- It is mistakenly presumed that chlorine foam can work both as cleaning and disinfecting agent
- Based on pH, hypochlorous acid (HOCl) molecule and the hypochlorite ion (OCl^-) are in equilibrium in chlorine solution
- Hypochlorous acid molecule (HOCl) is the chief biocidal present in chlorine releasing agents
- It is not charged and therefore, it is said that, it is able to pass through the microbial cell walls
- Chlorine releasing agents are prepared in the solution having pH 10–11
- So, the chlorine is largely present as the hypochlorite ion OCl^- at pH 10–11 which works fundamentally both as detergent and oxidising

agent, and thereby assist in removing proteins and grease and help in bleaching

- The effect of pH and dearth of free HOCl turns the chlorine solutions into weaker disinfectant (by hundred times) compared to simple hypochlorite disinfectant solution without any alkalis
- The improved cleaning action of the chlorine foam substantially eliminates bacterial load and dirt
- However, sensitivity to heat and light of chlorine renders residual bactericidal effect ineffective/short time

Non-oxidising disinfectants

- This class of disinfectants include quaternary ammonium compounds or 'quats' –cationic surfactants and amphoterics–class of surfactants having both positive and negative charges
- Stable to heat and less corrosive
- Having residual biocidal or biostatic effect
- These surfactant-based disinfectants are foaming which is problematic as it necessitates many rinsing cycles
- Or foaming can be advantageous as it enables visual inspection and procedural monitoring of the cleaning system

Disinfectants: its formulations and selection

- If disinfectants are not carefully formulated, it results in lower disinfection efficiency at low temperature or against few more hardy bacteria like *pseudomonads*
- Properly formulated disinfectants use various biocidal constituents along with surfactants and other agent to enhance its patency
- Well planned formulation too aids in eradicating the resistance development in microbes
- Development of resistance to various biocides and disinfectants is generally not found in factories such as food plant
- Disinfectants can be influenced by the detergents residues remaining on surfaces due to inefficient rinsing
- The cationic surfactant 'quats' can lose its effectiveness due to neutralization by the anionic surfactants present in the detergent
- Disinfectants selection should be in the consultation with the supplier as the material of surfaces to be disinfected, amount of soil residue suspected to be present after cleaning, workers and products safety, particular

microbes to be targeted, the surrounding and solution temperature and the duration of effect required (fast/residual effects) are to be considered

- In few instances, cleaning and disinfection processes may be joined together into one process using a sanitizer which acts both as detergent and disinfectant *eg.* quat- or amphoteric-based neutral or slightly alkaline compound
- Efficacy of disinfectants *i.e.* effects of biocidal molecule or designed disinfectant and to measure the minimum inhibitory concentration (MIC) of the each biocidal molecules or disinfectant formulation are assessed by disinfection assessment tests
- The MIC is the least concentration of an antimicrobial agent at which it will inhibit the growth of a particular microbial

Equipments related to cleaning & hygiene and application methods

There are various ways to apply detergents and disinfectants depending on the nature of the cleaning work

1. **Manual cleaning**
2. **Foam cleaning**
3. **Gels**
4. **Spray**
5. **Fogging**
6. **Cleaning-in-place (CIP)**

1. Manual cleaning

- In this method, the agents are applied manually with the help of cloth, mop, brush, pad, *etc.*
- Normally, it is restricted for small machinery or a particular area of a large machinery that are not water-resistant or which requires dismantling
- Labour exhaustive and can be unsafe if sharp or heavy equipment is involved
- Detergents or sanitizers (mixture of detergents–disinfectants) may be applied in this way but usually, disinfectants is not used

2. Foam cleaning

- Foam is generated with the help of equipment and is sprayed from a nozzle and left to act for normally 15-30 min
- Later, the loosened scales are removed by rinsing

- Foam cleaning is appropriate for big areas like floors, walls, stands, conveyors and tables and complex machinery like fillers, defeatherers, blackscrapers, *etc.*
- The foams only function as the carrier of detergents to act on the intended surfaces
- Creamy consistency of foam is considered the best quality foam compared to too dry or too wet
- The foam is sprayed as a thin, uniform coat
- Coverage rate is very high and largely economical
- A great volume of foam can be created from small quantity of detergent (up to 500-times)

Equipments for foam and disinfectant application

These equipments can be categorized as:

A. Mobile foam systems
B. Centralised foam systems
C. Satellite foam systems

A. Mobile foam systems

- Works with air-driven pumps and having tank injectors joined to high or medium pressure mobile washers

Advantages

- Reduced capital price and high flexibility
- Helps in applying various cleaning agents in different places of the plant

Disadvantages

- Controlling the chemicals concentration is difficult
- Maintenance of parts linked with movement of system hard
- Likely chance of wastage of unutilized solution

B. Centralised foam systems

- A system comprising one central automatic chemical dilution tank and one solution pump is used and liquid is forced under low pressure to various outlets set up on the pipe system spread all over the plant
- Compressed air is introduced into the outlet 'foam boxes' to produce the foam of the required flow rate and air content

Advantages

- One single central control on the chemical strength for whole area of plant
- Manual handling of concentrated chemicals is avoided
- No need to bring large quantity of chemicals inside the factory processing areas
- Chemicals quantity required is reduced by 10–20% compared to mobile tank foam system due to wastage reduction

Disadvantages

- Capital cost is more
- Decline of the diluted detergent solution within the system due to changes in the water quality

C. Satellite foam and disinfection systems

- Under this system, centralised rinse systems work through foam boxes installed on wall or trolley and fitted with venture injectors at each outlet
- In low- and medium-pressure rinse systems (about 20–40 bar water pressure) utilising multi-injector satellite stations, compressed air can be selectively applied at each injector to create detergent foam and disinfectant spray or foam
- In high-pressure rinse systems (>70 bar), only atmospheric air can be drawn in using special venturi foam lances.
- High-pressure fixed systems are now rarely been used

Advantages

- Low capital and running costs (dependent on existing systems)
- Full flexibility of choosing chemical /its level at each outlet
- Safe and easy for workers

Disadvantages

- Chemical drums have to kept in the processing areas

3. Gels

- Gel are produced using distinctive chemicals and spray equipment to provide a thick, and viscous coat of detergent that sticks powerfully to even vertical sides
- Sprayed on particular small areas where long contact time is required such as burnt/stubborn deposits

- Costly if applied in routine manner for larger areas of plant
- Longer contact time is needed
- Through rinsing of gels is problematic

4. Sprays

- In this, a gun and/or lance is attached to a pressurised water system and the disinfectant is introduced through an injector
- Because of foam cleaning technology, it is now seldom used
- Much wastage of cleaning agent in this method
- Tough to visualise the disinfectant application
- It is slower and inferior in performance to foam cleaning

5. Fogging

- Pressurized air is used to produce very fine mist of disinfectants which remain suspended in the air for long duration in the intended plant to give its effect and then settle down on the surfaces
- Thus, creating too small droplets (10–20 μm) and saturating the air with it will cause suspension of these droplets for long duration and thus, producing very good result
- Inability to produce mist of proper size and volume will result in disinfection of only upper surfaces of the plant due to quick settling down of the larger and weightier mists
- The main aim of the fogging is the whole surface disinfection in a designated closed area by aerosol
- Maximum benefits of fogging can be exerted if the earlier cleaning procedures were carried out correctly

6. Cleaning-in-place (CIP)

- CIP is widely used in liquid processing plants such as dairy for cleaning of the internal surfaces of the pipes, vessels, tankers, heat exchangers *etc.*
- CIP involves a programmed cycle, including pre-set timed pre-rinse, cleaning and rinsing stages
- CIP is automated or semi-automated with a system of valves, pumps and detergent tanks, controlled by microprocessor

The major factors to be considered in CIP are

i. Flow velocity
ii. Spray pressure and pattern
iii. Temperature
iv. Detergent contro
v. Chemical energy and foam control
vi. Recycling

i. Flow velocity

- It must be adequate in all parts of the system to produce turbulent movement of disinfectants
- Normally, it is near to 1.5–2 m/s—flow rate
- If the pipes diameters are different in the same system, the highest diameter pipe must have this flow rate
- Failure to achieve this flow rate will result in 'laminar' flow of the disinfectants at the edge near to the pipe surface having very small or no mechanical energy to aid in the cleaning

ii. Spray pressure and pattern

- For cleaning of interior surfaces of large tankers and vessels, spray balls or rotating jets are applied
- If the impact energy of the spray is not adequate or not able to reach the blind spots of the tanker/vessels, cleaning will be ineffective
- In low-pressure system, 1–3 bar and in high-pressure systems, 6 bar pressure is used
- 20–35 L/min/m is the required flow rate at the circumference of the vessels to have effective cleaning

iii. Temperature

- For highly effective rate of cleaning reactions, 70–85 °C solution temperature is usually used

iv. Detergent control

- Conductivity probe and pump based on temperature compensation controls the detergent supply in CIP System
- Conductivity minutely tracks the free caustic levels in CIP solutions and accordingly, automatically controls the flows of detergents in CIP system

- However, in manual dosing, there is danger that the chemical concentration may become too high or low

v. Chemical energy and foam control

- Generally, caustic based alkali detergents are chiefly used in CIP system
- Extra constituents may be added to the detergent to enhance its efficiency, for example, to prevent foaming and assist in wetting, surfactants are added, to dislodge deposits, chelating agents (*eg.* calcium phosphate) are added and such detergents are called built detergents
- Such additives are principally better and cost-effective, however, it need separate dose pumps for caustic detergents and additives

vi. Recycling of detergent solutions

- Detergent solutions may be used more number of times
- It is cost-effective and ecologically friendly and decreases the burden on effluent plants
- Reuse of solutions is based on the dirt quantity taken by the solution in each circulating cycle and on the chelating capacity of the detergent
- Detergent solution might deposit the scales again in the moving part of the system if the solution was already highly laden with soils and scales
- To wards off such problem, filtration or centrifugation is performed so that solution can be re-used many times

Rinse systems

- Meat plants need effective rinse systems for washing down the plant before and after the foam application and in some cases for generating the foam itself and applying disinfectant
- Proper rinse system is required in meat plants for washing foams pre and post foam application
- Also to create foam and apply disinfectant, rinse system is needed

There are three types of rinse systems:

i. Low-pressure water systems (pressure <10 bar)
ii. High-pressure rinse systems (pressure 60–120 bar)
iii. Medium-pressure rinse systems (pressure 20–40 bar)

i. Low-pressure (pressure <10 bar) water systems

- Insufficient for cleaning and rinsing meat or poultry processing plants due to absence of adequate energy in the water jet

ii. High-pressure (60–120 bar) rinse systems

- It is dependent on either built-in pump systems or movable pressure washers
- Use is declining--- due to maintenance, safety and hygiene basis
- System works at 60–120 bar with the help of piston pumps or plunger-type pumps
- Produce vibration in plumbed-in systems
- The water breaks up into fine droplets at almost 1 m losing its impact energy of water jet once it come out of nozzle due to the high velocity of the water
- So, rinsing of surfaces must be done from close distance

iii. Medium-pressure rinse systems (20–40 bar)

- System created to bring balance between pressure and volume
- It employs multistage centrifugal pumps and wider-bore, medium-pressure-rated pipe work and thus, does not produce vibration

Water temperatures

- Although, for knife sterilisation, water temperature of 82 °C is required as per the EU regulations but such higher temperatures are not practical for many meat plant cleaning process barring CIP
- Hence, the agreeable temperature is 50–65°C which is both effective and economical, and also liquefy the fats encountered in meat plants

Automated cleaning system

i. Cleaning-in-place system
ii Central cleaning system
iii. Self Contained system

i. Cleaning-in-place system

- Already discussed above
- Mainly used in dairy industry or industry handling liquids
- Limited use in meat plant

ii Central cleaning system (CCS)

- Involves a central pumping system which supplies the pressurized cleaning solutions all over the meat plant
- Flow rate of 136-181 lts./min is maintained under 35-49 kg/cm^2 of pressure

- In one type of CCS, detergents are mixed with water centrally and then supplied to different locations of the plant by single pipe. Later, plain water is used for ringing
- In another type of CCS, detergent is transported to different locations of the plant through one pipe and at each locations, it is mixed with high pressure water coming from another pipe and then used through a cleaning gun--- more costly

iii. Self-contained system

- Pumping source and chemical spray systems are contained in one unit
- Many small units are used in the same plants at different required locations depending on the need
- May be using hot water or steam
- Use acid cleaner or alkaline cleaner and sanitizer at each remote location of a plant
- Flexible system, if pump of one unit fails, a unit from another area can be used.

Sanitizing agents

- Sanitizer or disinfectants are applied only after thorough cleaning
- Coal tar preparation (phenol, cresol *etc.*) are not used in meat industry because of their strong smell
- Detergents followed by sanitizer application or a combination of both is required in meat processing plant under not less than 14 kg/cm^2 pressure and 82 °C solution temperature

The sanitizing agents fall into four main categories

i. Halogen-based formulations
ii. Quaternary ammonium compounds (QAC)
iii. Amphoteric compounds
iv. Acids & Alkalis
v. Tego compounds

i. Halogen-based formulations

- Chlorine is extensively applied in food industry as sanitizing agent or disinfectant
- Chlorine is manufactured as gas or hypochlorite solution

- When chlorine is dissolved in water, it forms hypochlorous acid and hypochlorite ions
- The ratio of these two depends on the pH of the solution and more hypochlorous acid is produced at low pH of the solution
- Hypochlorous acid has more sanitizing effect than hypochlorite ions
- The concentration required for abattoir sanitation is 130-220 ppm
- The maximum concentration required for carcase washing is 100 ppm
- 250 ppm of chlorine contained in sodium hypochlorite solution is applied on clean surfaces for disinfection
- Chlorine is little corrosive for metal especially at high temperature
- Chlorine gets inactive in the presence of organic matter

ii. Quaternary ammonium compounds (QAC)

- Are cationic detergents, good cleaning agent but not dependable disinfectant
- Bacteriostatic in nature ---mainly effective against Gram-positives
- Inactivated by the presence of organic matter
- Less corrosive to metal
- Hard water reduces QAC efficiency
- More expensive than halogens
- Cannot be mixed with anionic detergents such as soap

iii. Amphoteric compounds

- Are either long chain substituted amino acids or betaines
- Surface-active, compatible with all other detergents and sanitizers
- Not affected by hard water

iv. Acids & alkalis

- Strong mineral acids and caustic alkalis, boric acid, organic benzoic acid
- Rarely used in abattoirs for cleaning/sanitization
- Only used in special disinfection requirement

v. Tego compounds

- Are ampholytic derivatives of dodecyldi (aminoethyl) glycine and are surface active and bacteriostatic
- Inactivated by presence of hard water and organic matter
- Non-toxic but expensive

The cleaning sequence of a food plant

The ideal sequence for normal routine surface cleaning of a meat plant is:

1. Gross clean/preparation
2. Pre-rinsing
3. Application of detergent
4. Post-rinsing
5. Disinfection
6. Terminal rinsing

1. Gross clean/preparation

- Usually, this step is carried out utmost improperly or is totally overlooked
- Small fragments of meat, food items *etc.* bigger than fingernail are cleaned prior to detergent employment
- Cleaning process is negatively affected by the food particles remaining on the floors, surfaces and equipments as:
    - It guards surfaces and the bacteria on them from the detergent action
    - It counteracts and hinders the detergent resulting in lower action and wastage
    - It harbours bacteria --- source of recontamination
    - The left over grease and protein on the surfaces function as nutrient source for microbials and as an obstacle to disinfectant
    - It can be carried into the drainage system causing blockage in traps or can increase the biological oxygen demand (BOD) of the effluent
    - It inclines the cleaning workers to leave the areas unattended and not to check the effectiveness of the cleaning work
- An improper gross cleaning is the most important cause of variable surface bacterial counts and high bacterial contamination in air-droplets produced by rinsing

2. Pre-rinsing

- The main aim of the pre-rinsing is to remove the deposits which are difficult to be taken out by picking/scraping/shovelling
- It is essential in the cleaning of cutting boards having high fat/grease deposited inside the grooves and crevices of the boards making the real cleaning very difficult
- For pre-rinsing of fresh blood, the water temperature should be less than 50 °C to prevent coagulation

3. Application of detergent

- The main aim of the detergent application is to clean the surfaces of tough coating of protein, fat (grease) *etc.* which appears clean
- Detergents are not formulated for getting rid of big particles of meat or heavy fat coating
- Foam application must be systematic and full enveloping all the areas
- In foaming, its thickness, concentration, dryness and contact time (15–30 min) are more crucial

4. Post-rinsing

- Post-ringing is performed with caution to reduce the splash and aerosol formation as this would re-contaminate the areas or carry dirt to high up on the walls
- The surfaces should be absent from observable dirt, soils and detergent residues and should appear clean after post-rinsing
- Accumulated water should be removed from the surfaces and vessels after post-rinsing

5. Disinfection

- Surfaces to be disinfected should appear clean, rinsed well, devoid of any left over water
- Surfaces coming in contact with food should be disinfected minimum once in a day
- The concentration of the disinfectant and its contact time (ideally >20 minutes) are both very important.
- Concentration and contact time (preferably >20 min) are more crucial

6. Terminal rinsing

- Some disinfectants are formulated to be left on the surfaces without end rinsing and thus, creating residual level of disinfectant on surfaces
- Post-cleaning, this residual disinfectant keep a lower bacterial count for substantial period of time
- Besides, it give extra time for surfaces to dry as there is no need for terminal rinsing
- If terminal rinsing is needed, adequate time is given for surfaces to dry before the plant commences work
- Terminal rinsing is performed in lesser time compared to pre-rinsing and post-rinsing as no food particles/dirt is present

Monitoring of hygiene

Monitoring of cleaning and disinfection efficiency is performed by

1. *Visual assessment*
2. *Surface analysis and microbiology*

Rapid surface hygiene tests

- Rapid surface hygiene tests provide results in real time enabling quick decision to be taken regarding cleaning whether it is satisfactory or needs to be repeated
- These tests are normally dependent on the measurement of adenosine triphosphate (ATP)
- Food particles and microbes have abundant ATP and through swabs and reagents, these ATPs are picked up and reacted with luciferin–luciferase resulting in light emission. This process is called ***bioluminescence***
- The intensity of these emissions are measured by luminometers reflecting the ATP concentration and in turn, the level of food particles and microorganisms on the surface
- The fact that ATP test do not discriminate between somatic cells (from meat/food product) and microbial cells is almost immaterial, as it indicates the efficacy of whole cleanliness and microbial load (whether dead or live)

Microbiological assessment

- Microbiological tests should be done along with rapid hygiene tests to assess the cleaning process
- Microbiological assessment is crucial to keep checks on pathogenic and spoilage microorganisms
- The biodegradability of the detergents and disinfectants is significant--adds immensely to the effluent total COD/BOD
- Surfactants, alkylphenol ethoxylates (APEOs), is said to impart oestrogenic effects in river waters and may be influencing the reproduction of aquatic creatures

Odour control

Odour is released from the effluent plant if

- Aeration is insufficient
- loading is too much
- Anaerobic bacteria are thriving

Problems can be overcome by

- High aeration
- Decreasing the COD/BOD level of the meat plant
- Aiding the degradation of proteins and other organics materials by mixing enzyme formulation in the effluent water

17

Working of Effluent Treatment Plant (ETP)

Pollution emanating from industrial units has become a major problem globally and it is generally monitored by some government agencies. These agencies enforce various laws and regularly carry out checks at the industrial units. Same is true with regards to slaughterhouses or abattoirs. Pollution parameters are parameters against which the effluents coming out of the Effluent Treatment Plant (ETP) of slaughterhouse or any industrial entity is measured against. Effluent generated during various processes of the slaughterhouse is directed towards the ETP and it undergoes different processes to reduce the pollutants level in the effluent. Then, the effluent is tested against the pollution parameters and the effluent must have less than the maximum permissible level of the pollution parameters. The effluent must not have more than the permissible maximum level of the pollutants after coming out of ETP before being discharged into the municipal sewage system or some natural water bodies.

Pollution parameters are

1. Biochemical oxygen demand (BOD)
2. Chemical oxygen demand (COD)
3. Chloride (Cl)
4. Dry matter (DM) or total solids (TS)
5. Grease, fat and oil
6. pH
7. Total nitrogen (N)
8. Pathogenic bacteria
9. Suspended solids (SS)
10. Temperature
11. Turbidity and colour
12. Volatile solids (VS)

Pollution parameters

1. Biochemical oxygen demand (BOD)

- BOD is the quantity of the biodegradable organic matter present in the effluent
- A known volume of the effluent is mixed with a known volume of oxygen-saturated water and incubated at 20 °C for 5 days and the volume of oxygen consumed by the aerobic organisms is called as BOD level of the effluent wastewater
- It provides a measure of the concentration of pollutants in the effluent water

2. Chemical oxygen demand (COD)

- COD is quantity of the oxygen consumed for the oxidation of all oxidisable organic and inorganic matters in a known volume of effluent measured using chemical procedure
- Quicker and more precise ways of measuring the oxygen requirements of an effluent before directing it to ETP
- COD value provides a prognostic value of BOD
- The major difference between BOD and COD is that the BOD is measure of the oxygen demand of microorganisms present in the effluent water to oxidize organic matters available in the effluent under aerobic conditions whereas the COD is the oxygen required to chemically oxidize all the pollutants (organic + inorganic) presents in the effluent

Table 17.1 Differences between BOD and COD

S. No.		BOD	COD
1	**Definition**	Measure of oxygen consumed by the microorganisms present in effluent in oxidizing only the organic matter	Measure of oxygen required to oxidise both organic and inorganic matters present in the effluent
2	**Materials broken down**	Only organic matter	Both organic and inorganic matters
3	**Breakdown of organic matter**	Done by aerobic microorganisms	Done by chemical reagents in lab
4	**Complete breakdown of pollutants**	Does not take place	Takes place
5	**Strong oxidizing reagents**	No	Yes
6	**Time taken**	Normally nakes 5 days	Takes only few hours
7	**Value**	Lower than COD	Higher than BOD

3. Chloride (Cl)

- Salinity is measured by chloride content of the effluent

4. Dry matter (DM) or total solids (TS)

- It is the amount of weight obtained after drying the known weight of effluent at 105 °C for 24 h and expressed as g per litre or milligram per litre

5. Grease, fat and oil

- They are not soluble in water (immiscible in water)
- These materials form a layer on the various parts of ETP systems
- Tend to clog pipes, pumping systems and screens (sieves)
- Forms a coat on the top of effluent and thus, hinders oxygen transfer and therefore, jeopardises the working of aerobic digestion systems
- Results in foul odour as the deposited fat and oil turns rancid

6. pH

- Acidic or alkaline character of an aqueous solution is expressed in pH
- ETP system functions well at around neutral pH 7.0

7. Total nitrogen (N)

Total nitrogen (N) is found in 3 different forms in the wastewater:

i. Organic nitrogen

ii. Inorganic nitrogen and free ammonia and

iii. Nitrites

- Solution form of ammonia is poisonous to water flora and fauna: the maximum permissible level in effluent is 40 mg/L
- Elevated level of nitrate in natural water bodies promote algal and other plant proliferation (eutrophication) and results in choking of water flow and insufficient O_2 to aquatic lives
- The maximum permissible level of nitrate in potable water is 0.5 mg/L
- If the concentration is 0.5 mg/L or more and the water to which it is discharged is chlorinated water, it results in development of bad taste and foul odour as well as it leads to formation of THMs or trihalomethanes (a bio-cumulative and carcinogenic compound)

8. Pathogenic bacteria

- Coliform should be absent in potable water

9. Suspended solids (SS)

- SS shows the matters which are not soluble and remains in suspension in water
- Do not settle down or come at the top of the effluent
- Consist of both organic and inorganic materials

10. Temperature

- The effluent water when it is treated in ETP and then discharged in any natural body must have temperature equal or little higher than the temperature of the receiving water body as it would not affect the aquatic life

11. Turbidity and colour

- Treated effluent must be clear and colourless

12. Volatile solids (VS)

- Its quantity indicates biogas emission (not relevant to aerobic digestion, only related to anaerobic digestion)

Few important points

- The higher the BOD level of the effluent water, greater is the quantity of the organic matter and the higher is the pollution capacity of the effluent water
- Compared to domestic sewage (BOD 250-300 mg/litre), the effluents from the meat processing plant will have BOD level of 1500-2000 mg/litre
- Final waste load (animal tissue *etc.*) in the effluent water should be lower than 7.5 kg per 500 kg live weight slaughtered before treatment
- Water use should be lower than 5000 litres per 500 kg live weight slaughtered and BOD level of effluent should not exceed 1500 mg/kg before treatment

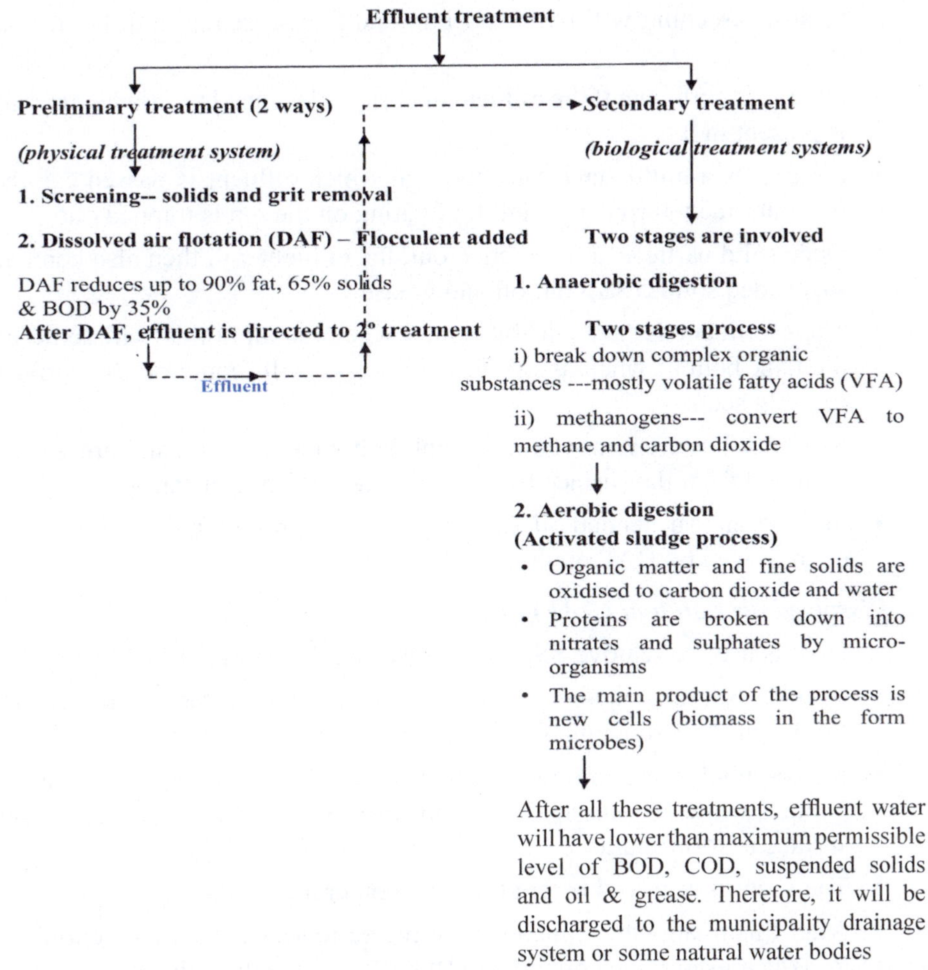

I. Preliminary treatment: performed in two steps (physical way)

i. Screening-- solid and grit removal using sieves of different diameters

- Preliminary treatment is the elimination of solids particles from the effluent
- Effluent are passed through different sieves/screens having different diameters
- Screens should be:
  - Non-clogging and self-cleaning
  - Adjustable to different water flow rates
  - Simple to clean either mechanically or manually
  - Odourless and noiseless

- Coarse screening will be 10–25 mm and fine screening will be to 5–6 mm
- Fat trap is sufficient if the effluent quantity is less and low-grade material is present in it
- Fat trap is a multi-stage tank through which effluent is passed calmly without much turbulence and fat floating on the top is trapped out
- Once solid particles are screened out, the effluent will then also contain suspended solids (SS), fat, oil and grease
- Then, effluent is taken in big tanks where small solids will settle at the tank bottom whereas oil, fat and grease will come on the surface forming scum
- Settled solids are removed from tank bottom and oil, fat and grease are removed from the surface by scrubber mechanism constantly
- Still, SS and suspended oil, fat and grease are present in the effluent and are removed by DAF method

ii. Dissolved air flotation (DAF) method

- DAF is used to remove SS, fats, grease and thus, lower BOD level
- In DAF, SS, fats, oil and grease are brought to the surface of the tank to form scum by producing micro-bubbles at the tank bottom
- Micro-bubbles are produced mechanically using pump and micro-bubbles while coming up on the top surface bring SS and oil on the top surface to form scum
- The scum is removed by continuous scraper mechanism
- After this treatment, effluents are directed to secondary treatment plant to reduce its organic content and BOD to an acceptable level
- DAF reduces 90% fat, 65% solids and BOD by 65%

Flocculants addition

- Mixing chemicals that help in flocculation (more bubbles formation) helps in removal of higher amount of BOD, SS and fat
- Flocculants like ferric chloride/sulphate, ferrous sulphate, aluminium sulphate (alum), sodium carbonate (soda ash), calcium carbonate (lime), polyelectrolytes and others are added to the effluent water
- Every flocculent functions at an ideal pH range
- And so, the pH of the effluent water is altered according to the optimal pH of the flocculent used

- Normally, caustic soda or hydrochloric acid is used to modify the effluent pH

Table 17.2: BOD values of few animal products processing plants

S. No.	Animal products processing plants	BOD (mg/l)
1.	Poultry processing plant	1000–1200
2.	Pig meat plant	1500–2000
3.	Large ruminants/sheep meat processing plant	1400–3200
4.	Fish processing plant	1000–3000
5.	Dairy (washings) plant	600–1300

II. Secondary treatment: performed in two steps

i. Anaerobic digestion

ii. Aerobic digestion

- In secondary treatment---biological treatment systems are used (microorganisms are used)
- In this treatment, favourable conditions for microbial growth is maintained and microbes consume the organic matter present in the effluent for their own cell synthesis and during this process, organic matters are degraded

i. Anaerobic digestion

- Anaerobic conditions are provided by carrying out this reaction in air tight tank
- There is quick degradation of organic material releasing biogas (CH_4)
- This system is more beneficial if the BOD lever is more than 2000 mg/l
- Tanks 4.5 m deep and loaded to 7.5 kg BOD per 5000 litres pond volume (*i.e.* BOD value 1500 mg/ litre) will give a BOD reduction of 60-80% at 30-32 °C
- In this digestion, two stage fermentations take place which occur concurrently

Two stages of anaerobic digestion

a) In the first stage, organic compounds are degraded into more simpler compounds by the microbials and volatile fatty acids (VFA) is one of the most important compound formed

b) In the second stage, this VFA is further broken down into methane and carbon dioxide by methanogenic bacteria

ii) Aerobic digestion (Activated sludge process)

- Aerobic digestion is more resistant to shock loading and the reaction time is shorter and hence, the tanks are small in size and low-priced
- On the bottom of the digester tank, air is pumped in using low-pressure air blowers or via surface aerators using electric motor so that micro-bubbles are produced for adding oxygen creating aerobic condition
- The level of required oxygenation depends on the level of dissolved oxygen, retention time and effluent-loading rate, pH, temperature, presence of toxic substances, organic content and discharge rate
- Keeping the pH at near 7.0–7.2 is very crucial
- Too much VFA production should be controlled as it will decrease the pH and the whole process will end
- Since, new microbial cell are synthesized, it is a 'living' process and effluent addition should be balanced
- Blood is not allowed to be mixed with effluent as it will increase the BOD level too much and the excess protein will stop the process
- Shallow ponds 0.9- 1.2 m deep having a loading of 7.3-9.1 kg BOD per day per hectare of pond surface are effective
- The suspended organic matter, colloidal particles and other solids are oxidised to carbon dioxide and water
- Proteins are degraded into nitrates and sulphates by various mixture of microbes
- After the reaction is over, the effluent is divided into two; supernatant which is clear water and settled solids which is called sludge containing new microbial cells (biomass)
- The most important result of the process is new microbial cells (biomass)
- A small portion of this sludge having biomass (active bacteria) along with other materials which were not degraded are taken out from the digester and used for oxidation of the next batch of incoming effluent
- This small portion of sludge containing active microbes are essential to maintain the aerobic degradation process of organic matters in the effluent
- The supernatant liquid is discharged into the sewage system or additionally, treated if needed
- The remaining sludge (waste activated sludge) is taken out and centrifuged to separate the water and the solid is dried/incinerated and disposed as fertilizer

Different types of aerobic digestion system

1. Oxidation Ditch System

- Developed by Dr. A. Pasveer in Holland (1953)
- One stage process of purification by aerobic digestion
- Oxidation of influent done by aeration rotor
- Sludge formed is oxidized to great extent--- finally, sludge is dried and further used as fertiliser

Actual Process

- The waste water flows into the aeration tank and it is mixed with earlier formed sludge
- The mixer moves to next tank and oxidation takes place
- Microbes break down the organic matter
- Finally, a portion of settled sludge is returned to the first tank
- Process continues like this

2. Biological Filtration Processes

It has two forms:

i. Percolating or trickling filters

ii Plastic-packed filters

i. Percolating or trickling filters

- Consists of 1.8-2.4 m beds of stone 50-100 mm diameter
- Purification done by films of microbes formed over the stones- oxidation of organic matters
- With a loading of 75-87 kg BOD per 5000 litres of packing per day, a BOD reduction of 40% is achieved

Disadvantages of this system

- Tendency to be blocked
- High capital cost
- Large land area required

ii Plastic-packed filters

- Developed to overcome the disadvantages of the percolating filters
- Higher loading of 115-125 kg BOD per 5000 litres of packing --- BOD reduction of 75-95% is achieved
- Expected reduction of BOD, SS and NH_3 in influent waste water after undergoing through waste water treatment

Table 17.3. Standards for discharge of effluents from slaughterhouses, meat processing plants and sea food industry

Industry	Various parameters of effluent coming out of plants	Standard (Maximum permissible levels are in mg/l except for pH)
Slaughterhouses/ meat processing units or both	pH	6.5 to 8.5
	Biochemical Oxygen demand (BOD) (3 days at 27 °C)	30
	Chemical Oxygen demand (COD)	250
	Suspended solids	50
	Oil and grease	10
Sea food industry	Biochemical Oxygen demand (BOD) (3 days at 27 °C)	30
	Suspended solids	50
	Oil and grease	10

Note: Revised standards for slaughterhouses notified on 28.10.2016 under the Environment (Protection) Rules 1986)

Index

Y

Z